CORE CLINICAL CASES

Self-assessment for Medical Students

Anatomy and Physiology

Learning by Modified Essay Questions

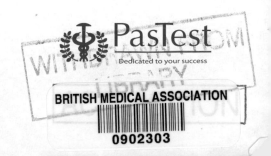

PasTest
Dedicated to your success

DEDICATION

To all friends at Glasgow University

CORE CLINICAL CASES

Self-assessment for Medical Students
Anatomy and Physiology

Marjorie E M Allison BSc MD, FRCP
Hon. Senior Research Fellow, Medical Education,
The Medical School, University of Glasgow

Stuart W McDonald BSc MB ChB PhD FRCS
Senior Lecturer in Anatomy, Laboratory of Human Anatomy
University of Glasgow

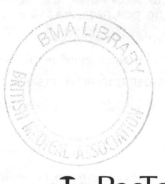
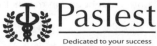
PasTest
Dedicated to your success

Egerton Court
Parkgate Estate
Knutsford
Cheshire
WA16 8DX

Telephone: 01565 752000

First Published 2008

ISBN: 1 905635 2 65

978 1 905635 2 69

A catalogue record for this book is available from the British Library.

The information contained within this book was obtained by the author from reliable sources. However, while every effort has been made to ensure its accuracy, no responsibility for loss, damage or injury occasioned to any person acting or refraining from action as a result of information contained herein can be accepted by the publishers or author.

PasTest Revision Books and Intensive Courses

PasTest has been established in the field of postgraduate medical education since 1972, providing revision books and intensive study courses for doctors preparing for their professional examinations.

Books and courses are available for the following specialties:

MRCGP, MRCP Parts 1 and 2, MRCPCH Parts 1 and 2, MRCS, MRCOG Parts 1 and 2, DRCOG, DCH, FRCA, PLAB Parts 1 and 2, Dentistry.

For further details contact:

PasTest, Freepost, Knutsford, Cheshire WA16 7BR

Tel: 01565 752000Fax: 01565 650264

www.pastest.co.uk   enquiries@pastest.co.uk

Text prepared by Carnegie Book Production, Lancaster

Printed and bound in the UK by CPI, Antony Rowe

CONTENTS

INTRODUCTION

We are grateful to PasTest for inviting us to write a book of modified essay questions (MEQs) in Anatomy and Physiology. We have interpreted these disciplines broadly to include neuroanatomy and development as well as important areas of pharmacology, biochemistry and immunology, without which the material presented would have been unbalanced. The format of the MEQs is similar to that used for summative assessment at the Medical School of the University of Glasgow. When this style of question was first introduced in the late 1960s it was intended to provide a means of assessing cognitive skills and reasoning, rather than simply recalling a list of 'facts'. To write such questions well is difficult and many MEQs, including ours, include much recall of factual knowledge. Only those questions that use terms such as 'why'' justify' or 'explain' will address reasoning skills.

In response to the General Medical Council's document *Tomorrow's Doctors*, medical curricula in the UK were redesigned, integrating medical science and clinical teaching. Such curricula contain the concept of a spiral of learning where topics recur, but in increasing depth and with more connections with other gathered information. We hope that students at all levels of undergraduate medical training will find the revision material useful but it is primarily aimed at students in the later years of their medical course.

A cohort of medical students in their final years wrote the patient-based scenarios. The material presented is thus largely what they felt their peers would find interesting, reflect core knowledge and be useful for revision. We wish to express our thanks to the students whose names are listed within. Without their assistance this project would never have come to fruition. The authors have edited the material to provide an appropriate balance and a more uniform style. They also added to it, where their experience suggested there were gaps, to provide a more comprehensive coverage. We make no apology for inclusion of common medical eponyms. Despite recent suggestions that eponyms are redundant they are widely used. 'Eponyms bring colour to medicine … they embed medical traditions and culture in our history.'(Whitworth, BMJ Sep 2007; 335:425).

We hope that medical students will enjoy working through the patient-based material and find the book helpful. The anatomical and physiological content reflects the authors' philosophy that a sound grasp of basic science is important in medical practice.

Marjorie E. Allison and Stuart W. McDonald, University of Glasgow, April 2008

ACKNOWLEDGEMENTS

We are extremely grateful to Mrs Cathy Dickens of PasTest who made the initial approach, co-ordinated the project, and who has shown endless understanding and patience in our many telephone and e-mail communications. It has been a great pleasure working with her. The invaluable help of Mrs Dicken's support staff who have set the type-face, produced the illustrations and proof-read the text is also most gratefully acknowledged.

CONTRIBUTORS

Thirty-three Fourth and Fifth Year medical students contributed significantly to the development of these questions. They participated in a Student Selected Module on Assessment. As part of this each had to submit a complete modified essay question for 30 marks on a subject of their choosing. The students were responsible for the scenario, the questions, answers and learning points. The authors were responsible for checking and editing these and for providing additional material as appropriate.

Tahir Akhtar

Mosaab Aljalahma

Colin Black

Margaret Cairns

Lauren Clarke

David Cowell

Fiona Ferguson

Gemma Fleming

Stuart Fraser

Anjuman Ghaznavi

Ciara Harris

Charlotte Heath

Susie Hewitt

Chistopher Ho Chong Teck

Sacha Haworth

Alesia Hunt

Julie Langan

Susan Lockhart

Subashini M

Euan Mabon

Louise McFadden

Judith McGhee

Gregg Miller

Andrew Mullett

Rachel Noble

Christine Obondo

Michelle Rae

Sonya Scott

Lisa Seerathun

Fiona Thorburn

Selina Tsim

Kok Loong Ue

Yao Yong

QUESTIONS

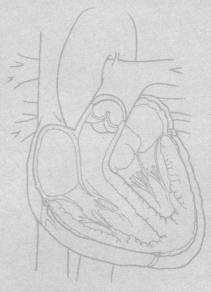

CARDIOLOGY CASES:
QUESTIONS

CARDIOLOGY
1. CONGENITAL HEART DISEASE

You are a junior doctor working in the Paediatric Accident and Emergency Department. Mrs Smith, a 32-year-old mother, presents with her 6-week-old baby, Jack. Mrs Smith says Jack has been sweating and increasingly breathless during his feeds over the past week or so. He has also been quite irritable over this period. Prior to this, Baby Jack was well and he was on the 50th centile for head circumference, length and weight. His neonatal examination was normal.

You examine Jack, and note he is tachypnoeic (60 breaths per minute), and tachycardic (170 beats per minute). He is not cyanosed, and there are no signs of upper airway obstruction, though there is slight wheeze and intercostal recession.

You auscultate Jack's precordium, listening for heart sounds and murmurs. You hear a loud pansystolic murmur at the lower left sternal edge with a split second heart sound. On listening to the chest, you hear scattered wheezes. From the history and examination, you suspect a congenital heart defect and arrange an ECG, chest X-ray and echocardiogram.

As you wait for the above investigations to be carried out, you revise the anatomy and physiology of the fetal circulation.

Q **1. Label the following diagram of the fetal circulation.** *4 marks*

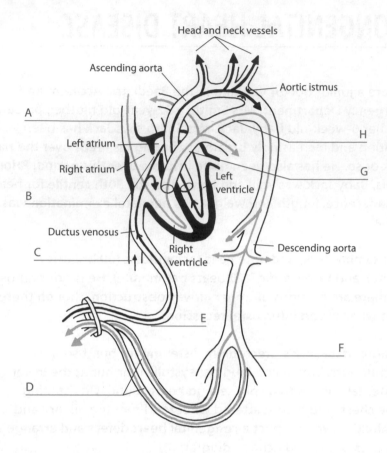

Figure 1.1: Anatomy of fetal circulation.

½ mark each:

A – _____

B – _____

C – _____

D – _____

E – _____

F –

G –

H –

Q 2. Please answer the following questions on the fetal circulation.   *4 marks*

Q 2(a). Through which opening does deoxygenated blood leave the fetal right atrium?

Q 2(b). In which organ does the ductus venosus lie?

Q 2(c). What does the umbilical vein become after birth?

Q 2(d). Which atrium of the heart, left or right, has the higher pressure in its chamber during fetal life?

You consider the development of the fetal heart, which initially forms as a tubular structure and is subsequently partitioned.

Q 3. At what age does the early heart begin to beat?   *1 mark*

Please look at the following diagram of the early heart.

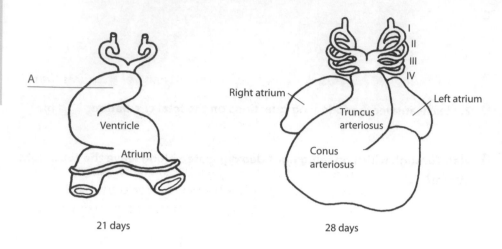

Figure 1.2: Anatomy of the early heart.

Q 4. Structure A is the outflow tract in the early embryonic heart. What is this structure commonly called? *1 mark*

Q 5. Which structures form from the truncus arteriosus, the distal part of structure A? *1 mark*

Q 6. Postganglionic sympathetic and parasympathetic neurons become associated with the developing heart. What is the embryological source of these ganglion cells? *1 mark*

Q 7. On the diagram of the fetal heart at 28 days, there are structures labelled
I–IV. What are these structures collectively known as?   *1 mark*

Q 8. Structures I–IV above eventually form various definitive structures. Name
two such adult structures that are derived from I–IV.   *1 mark*

The echocardiography report for Baby Jack becomes available,
and confirms a congenital heart lesion – a ventricular septal defect
(VSD). You consider how Baby Jack's symptoms can be explained by
this pathology.

Q 9. You first of all consider the normal pressures in the chambers of the *adult*
heart. Please complete the following table of pressures within the chambers
of the heart, using the options below. (Each option may be used once, more
than once, or not at all.)   *4 marks*

- <10 mmHg
- 25 mmHg
- 40 mmHg
- 80 mmHg
- 120 mmHg
- 180 mmHg

Chamber of heart	Blood pressure (mmHg)	
	Systolic	Diastolic
Right atrium		
Right ventricle		
Left atrium		
Left ventricle		

½ mark for each.

CARDIOLOGY

You recall, however, that the equivalent blood pressures in the neonate and infant are much lower than the adult values shown above.

Q 10. In what direction is blood flowing across Baby Jack's VSD?   *1 mark*

Q 11. At which part of the interventricular septum does a congenital defect most commonly occur?   *1 mark*

You recall that on auscultating Jack's precordium, you heard a loud pansystolic murmur at the lower left sternal edge with a fixed, split second heart sound.

Q 12. In general, what can you can deduce about the size of a VSD if it produces a loud murmur?   *1 mark*

Q 13. Explain why the murmur found in Baby Jack is pansystolic.   *1 mark*

Q 14. Explain why the fixed split second heart sound is produced in Baby Jack.   *2 marks*

Q 15. With reference to fetal circulation and changes in the cardiovascular system that occur in the weeks after birth, why has Baby Jack been asymptomatic with his VSD up until now, 6 weeks after birth? Why is he symptomatic now? *2 marks*

Q 16. You look at Baby Jack's chest X-ray and note that the cardiothoracic ratio is around 55%. Is this abnormal? *1 mark*

Q 17. Describe one other change you would expect to see on Baby Jack's chest X-ray. *1 mark*

You decide to treat Baby Jack with furosemide before referring him to the paediatric cardiologists for their opinion and possible surgery.

Q 18. With reference to cardiac workload, how would furosemide help with Baby Jack's symptoms? *2 marks*

CARDIOLOGY

📖 BIBLIOGRAPHY

Barnes N, Archer N. 2005. Understanding congenital heart disease. *Current Paediatrics*, **15,** 421–428.

Brown K. 2005. The infant with undiagnosed cardiac disease in the emergency department. *Clinical Pediatric Emergency Medicine*, **6**, 200–206.

Carlson B M. 2004. *Human Embryology and Developmental Biology*, 3rd edn. New York: Elsevier, p. 447

Julian D G, Cowan J C, McLenachan J M. 2005. *Cardiology*, 8th edn. London: Elsevier Saunders.

Lissauer T, Clayden G. 2007. *Illustrated Textbook of Paediatrics*, 2nd edn. Edinburgh: Mosby.

Moore K L, Persaud T V N. 2003. *The Developing Human: Clinically Orientated Embryology*, 7th edn. London: Saunders.

Newby D E, Grubb N R. 2005. *Cardiology: An Illustrated Colour Text*. London: Churchill Livingstone, p. 134.

CARDIOLOGY
2. DOWN SYNDROME AND CONGENITAL CARDIAC ABNORMALITIES

You are on call in paediatrics, when you are asked to visit Baby Taylor, a newborn baby on the maternity ward, for a 'baby check' examination. While carrying out your examination you notice some dysmorphic features, and you think that Baby Taylor may have Down syndrome[a].

Q 1. List six dysmorphic features, visible on inspection, which are commonly associated with Down syndrome. *3 marks*

Q 2. Name one neurological finding which is likely to be found on examination of Baby Taylor. *1 mark*

Q 3. What is the commonest genetic abnormality in Down syndrome? *1 mark*

You discover that Mrs Taylor is aged 42 years with a possible family history of Down syndrome. She was offered antenatal diagnostic tests but declined.

Q 4. What test would she have been offered? *1 mark*

Q 5. Approximately how common is Down syndrome in pregnancies where the mother is over 40 years of age: 1 in 25; 1 in 100; 1 in 1000; 1 in 10 000? *1 mark*

You report your suspicions to your consultant, who agrees with your diagnosis. On examination of Baby Taylor he also hears a heart murmur. He informs Mr and Mrs Taylor that he suspects their child has Down syndrome and that he would like to arrange some genetic tests. He also explains that some children with Down syndrome are at a higher risk of other medical problems, and that he is also going to arrange some tests to look at Baby Taylor's heart.

Q 6. What is the most appropriate investigation to visualise Baby Taylor's heart and its function? *1 mark*

Q 7. Apart from cardiac abnormalities, name one other structural congenital abnormality commonly associated with Down syndrome. *1 mark*

The investigations confirm that baby Taylor has a ventricular septal defect (VSD).

Q 8. Describe the type of murmur that will be heard in a VSD in terms of where in the cardiac cycle it occurs. *1 mark*

Q 9. What is an 'innocent murmur'? *1 mark*

The parents come to the paediatric cardiac clinic, with Baby Taylor, to discuss the diagnosis. Mr Taylor has been reading the patient information leaflet and also researching congenital heart disease on the Internet. He tells the consultant that he has been reading about 'blue babies' and asks if Baby Taylor will go blue.

Q 10. Name one cyanotic heart condition. *1 mark*

Q 11. Label this diagram of the fetal circulation. *4 marks*

½ mark each

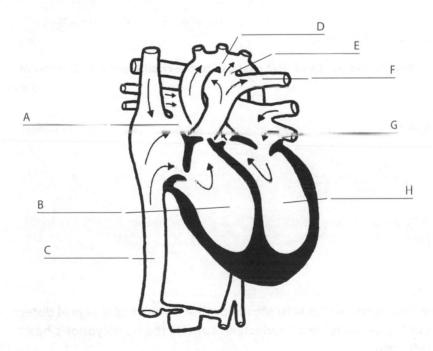

Figure 1.3: Fetal circulation.

A –

B –

C –

D –

E –

F –

G –

H –

Q 12. Explain the purpose of the ductus arteriosus.   *2 marks*

Q 13. Describe the physiological changes to the circulation which occur at birth.   *5 marks*

The consultant explains to Mr Taylor that a ventricular septal defect is not a 'blue baby' heart defect. It is one of the non-cyanotic heart conditions.

Q 14. The following are diagrams of non-cyanotic heart conditions.
Please name each condition.   *4 marks*

A

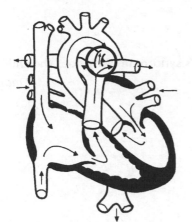

B

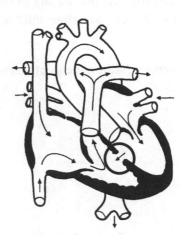

C

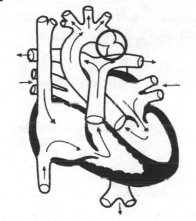

D

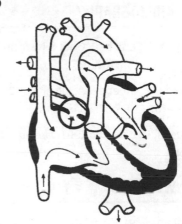

A –

B –

C –

D –

The consultant explains that if the VSD is not repaired, it could develop into a cyanotic or 'blue' syndrome in later life, a phenomenon known as Eisenmenger's[b] syndrome. He tells the Taylors that unfortunately in the past children with Down syndrome often did not have their VSD repaired.

Q 15. Explain pathogenesis of Eisenmenger's syndrome (Why does the child go blue?)

3 marks

Mr and Mrs Taylor decide to go ahead with the surgery.

📖 BIBLIOGRAPHY

Forrester C, Carachi R, Goel K N, Young D G. 1996. *Children's Medicine and Surgery*. London: Arnold.

Haddad D F, Greene S A, Olver R E. 2000. *Core Paediatrics and Child Health*. Edinburgh: Churchill Livingstone.

Lissauer T, Clayden G. 2001. *Illustrated textbook of Paediatrics*, 2nd edn. London: Mosby.

📖 WEBSITES

American Heart Association: www.americanheart.org

Down syndrome UK: www.downs-syndrome.org.uk

Women's Health Information www.womens-health.co.uk/downs.asp

[a]John Langdon Down (1828–1896), English physician noted for his work with mentally retarded children. He described the features of Down Syndrome in 1866.

[b]Victor Eisenmenger (1864–1932), Austrian physician who described Eisenmenger's syndrome in 1897. The term was coined by Dr Paul Wood in 1958.

CARDIOLOGY
3. VALVULAR HEART DISEASE AND EMBOLISM

You are the Foundation Year 2 House Officer and are receiving for the medical team. Mr Smith, a 69-year-old man, has been referred by his GP with a suspected ischaemic right foot. The foot pain came on earlier in the day. Mr Smith has been complaining of fatigue, general malaise and breathlessness over the past few weeks, which has been gradually increasing and is worse on exertion. He had a myocardial infarction 2 years ago and made an uneventful recovery.

On examination you find that Mr Smith's right foot is pale and cool but there is no ulceration of the skin. You check the peripheral pulses. As you palpate each pulse you picture the artery running close to the bone.

Q **1. For each of the pulses given in the table below, select the bony site with which it is most closely associated from the following list.** *3 marks*

Patella	Lateral malleolus
Lower femur	Calcaneus
Upper tibia	Talus
Head of fibula	Navicular
Shaft of tibia	Cuboid
Medial malleolus	

Pulse	Associated region of bone
Popliteal	
Posterior tibial	
Dorsalis pedis	

The femoral pulse is present on the right side but no more distal pulses are palpable. All the pulses are palpable on the left side.

Q 2. Which is the most likely artery to have been obstructed?   *1 mark*

You carry out a general examination of the patient. You note that Mr Smith's radial pulse is 168 bpm and is irregularly irregular.

Q 3. What is this heart rhythm?   *1 mark*

Q 4. Briefly outline the underlying electrical abnormality of the heart.
2 marks

Q 5. In patients with an irregularly irregular pulse, the pulse measured by auscultation of the apex beat is often faster than that measured at the radial pulse. What is this phenomenon called and explain why it happens?
2 marks

You now carry out a full examination of Mr Smith's cardiovascular system. On auscultation of the heart you hear a murmur. At this point you pause to review the cardiac cycle in order to help with your diagnosis.

Q 6. Here is a list of options of possible timings of events in the cardiac cycle relative to ventricular systole and diastole.

Option 1: Throughout ventricular systole

Option 2: Throughout ventricular diastole

Option 3: Early ventricular systole

Option 4: End of ventricular systole

Option 5: Early ventricular diastole

Option 6: End of ventricular diastole

Q In the table below give the timing option that best fits each event. The options may be used once, more than once, or not at all. *5 marks*

Event	Option
Flow into the ascending aorta	
Opening of aortic valve	
Closure of mitral valve	
Closure of tricuspid valve	
Flow through mitral valve	

You listen again to Mr Smith's heart and confirm that you have heard a systolic murmur. It is best heard at the apex and radiates towards the axilla.

Q 7. What is the definition of a murmur? *1 mark*

Q 8. The causes of systolic murmurs can be divided depending on whether they are ejection, pansystolic or late systolic. Insert the following causes of a systolic murmur into the appropriate lines in the table below. Each line in the answer box represents a different condition **3 marks.**

Aortic stenosis

Mitral regurgitation

Mitral valve prolapse

Pulmonary stenosis

Tricuspid regurgitation

Ventricular septal defect

Ejection	
Pansystolic	
Late systolic	

Q 9. Identify A–J on the following diagram (Figure 1.4). **5 marks**

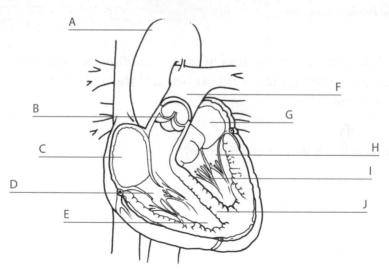

Figure 1.4: Anatomy of the heart.

A –

B –

C –

D –

E –

F –

G –

H –

I –

J –

You suspect that an embolus has formed and passed to the right lower limb. The Registrar sends for the on-call vascular surgeon. A Doppler ultrasound confirms the diagnosis. The surgeon plans to take Mr Smith to theatre to carry out an urgent embolectomy. The surgeon takes particular note of the time since the onset of the patient's foot symptoms. Had the ischaemia been prolonged he would have carried out fasciotomy, incision of the deep fascia bounding the osteofascial compartments of the lower limb. This is done to prevent muscular damage due to pressure caused by swelling of the contents of the compartments.

The diagram on the next page (Figure 1.5) shows a cross-section through the calf and the osteofascial compartments: anterior, peroneal, superficial posterior and deep posterior.

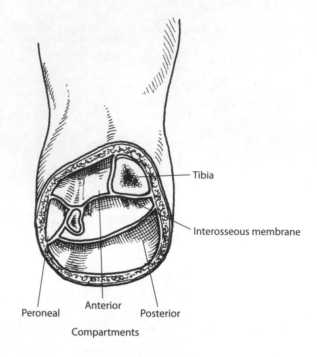

Figure 1.5: Cross-section through the calf and osteofascial compartments.

Q **10. In which compartment does each of the following muscles lie?** *5½ marks*

Extensor digitorum longus

Extensor hallucis longus

Flexor hallucis longus

Flexor digitorum longus

Gastrocnemius

Peroneus brevis (fibularis brevis)

Peroneus longus (fibularis longus)

Peroneus tertius (fibularis tertius)

Soleus

Tibialis anterior

Tibialis posterior

Anterior compartment	Peroneal compartment	Superficial posterior compartment	Deep posterior compartment

Q 11. Which nerve innervates the muscles in each of these compartments?

1½ marks

Anterior compartment	Peroneal compartment	Posterior compartment

📖 BIBLIOGRAPHY

Levick J R. 2000. *An Introduction to Cardiovascular Physiology*, 3rd edn. London: Arnold Publishers

Longmore M, Wilkinson I, Torok E. 2001. *Oxford Handbook of Clinical Medicine*, 5th edn. Oxford: Oxford University Press.

CARDIOLOGY
4. MYOCARDIAL INFARCTION

You are the house officer on duty one evening in the Accident and Emergency Department when a 46-year-old man, Mr Clark, is brought in at 21.30 hours by the paramedic team from his home because of severe crushing central chest pain. He has no previous history of ill health. The pain started suddenly at around 19.30 hours while he was watching TV. You suspect that he has suffered a myocardial infarction.

Mr Clark complains of nausea and has vomited. He also tells you that his chest pain is radiating to his jaw and down his left arm. On examination, he is sweating and cold. He has a tachycardia and is breathless.

The autonomic nervous system is likely to be responsible for some of the symptoms and signs.

Q 1. **Which division of the autonomic nervous system is likely to be responsible for the tachycardia, sweating and the cold peripheries?** *1 mark*

Q 2. **Which cranial nerves are likely to be responsible for the nausea and vomiting?** *1 mark*

Q 3. **Which spinal nerves have their dermatomes: (a) in the anterior part of the neck and (b) in the upper limb?** *2 marks*

a. **Anterior neck:**

b. **Upper limb:**

Q 4. Why does pain of cardiac origin radiate to the neck and to the upper limb? *4 marks*

Mr Clark has a 12 lead ECG carried out on arrival in the A & E Department.

A copy is shown in Figure 1.6.

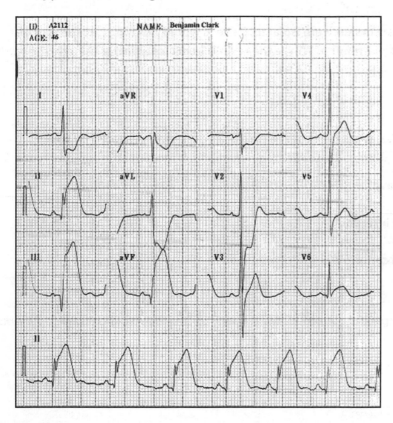

Figure 1.6: A 12-lead ECG.

Q 5. Calculate the heart rate. *1 mark*

Q 6. Mr Clark's ECG shows sinus rhythm. How can you tell? *2 marks*

Q 7. What is the pacemaker of the heart and where is it situated? *1 mark*

Q 8. If the pacemaker were isolated, its cells would discharge at the rate of about 100 per minute. Why is the resting heart rate slower than this? *1 mark*

Q 9. In an ECG, what parts of the cardiac cycle are represented by the following: *3 marks*

9(a). The P-wave?

9(b). The P-Q interval?

9(c). The QRS complex?

Q 10. What specific abnormalities are seen in the above ECG traces? *2 marks*

Q 11. What is the diagnosis?   *3 marks*

Q 12. Identify by name each of the labelled blood vessels A–H on the diagram of the anterior view of the heart (Figure 1.7).   *4 marks*

A –

B –

C –

D –

E –

F –

G –

H –

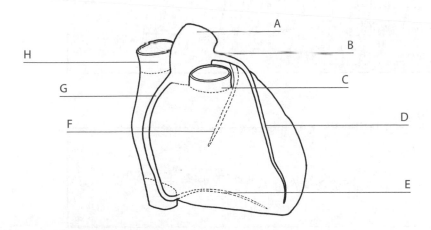

Figure 1.7: Anterior view of the heart.

Q 13. Identify on the diagram (with an X) the most likely site of arterial obstruction in this patient.   *1 mark*

Shortly after the first ECG, at approximately 21.50 hours, Mr Clark suddenly vomited, had what the nurse described as a 'seizure' and became unconscious with no palpable pulses.

Lead II of his ECG was recorded at this point (Strip A).

This was followed shortly by the onset of a different rhythm (Strip B).

Q 14. Name the rhythm shown in each ECG (Figure 1.8). What was the heart rate in strip A?   *3 marks*

Strip A

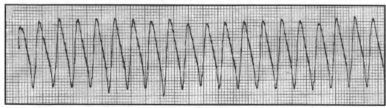

Strip B

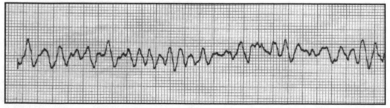

Figure 1.8: ECG.

Q 15. **What would be the principal means used to resuscitate Mr Clark at this point?** *1 mark*

📖 **BIBLIOGRAPHY**

Hampton J R. 2003. *The ECG Made Easy*, 6th edn. Edinburgh: Churchill Livingstone.

Kumar P, Clark M. 2005. *Clinical Medicine*, 6th edn. Edinburgh: Elsevier Saunders.

Williams P L. 1995. *Gray's Anatomy*, 38th edn. Edinburgh: Churchill Livingstone.

CARDIOLOGY
5. HEART FAILURE

You are the junior doctor on medical receiving on a busy Saturday night when you are called to the Accident and Emergency Department to see Mr Mayor, a 65-year-old retired teacher. Mr Mayor is gasping for breath, anxious and sweating. He is coughing up pink frothy sputum and on auscultation you hear crackling sounds, best heard as he breathes in. He is apyrexial. You diagnose acute pulmonary oedema and ask the nurses to ensure that he is kept sitting upright.

Q 1. List three treatments that you should give Mr Mayor at this stage. Include doses of any drugs.   *3 marks*

_____

_____

_____

Following your treatment, Mr Mayor is less breathless and you are able to take a more detailed history, carry out a thorough examination of the cardiovascular system and order necessary investigations. He tells you that he has had heart failure for the past 3 years following two myocardial infarctions in the past. He has smoked 20 cigarettes a day since he started teaching in his twenties.

You examine him carefully.

Q 2. List three symptoms and three signs of right and left heart failure in the table opposite.   *6 marks; ½ mark each*

	Right heart failure	Left heart failure
Symptoms		
Signs		

While you are arranging further investigations for Mr Mayor, the nurse hands you Mr Mayor's chest X-ray taken on admission.

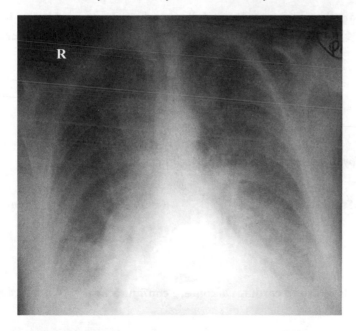

Figure 1.9: Mr Mayor's PA chest film.

Q 3. Give four characteristic features of heart failure that can be seen on this PA chest X-ray. *4 marks*

You arrange for Mr Mayor to be admitted to the cardiology ward for specialist care. The next morning the medical student on a cardiology placement approaches you after the ward round and asks you to clarify some concepts regarding heart failure.

You remind her of the equation used to determine cardiac output:

Cardiac output = heart rate × stroke volume

Q 4. List three factors that could result in a fall in stroke volume, and hence in cardiac output. *1 mark*

Q 5. The graph below illustrates the Frank[a]–Starling[b] Law.

Q 5(a). What is the Frank–Starling Law? *1 mark*

Q 5(b). How does this relate to cardiac sarcomere configuration? *1 mark*

Use the graph (Figure 1.10) and the above equation to answer the following questions.

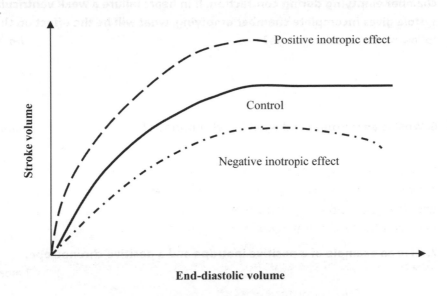

Figure 1.10: Relationship between end-diastolic volume and stroke volume.

Q **5(c). At a constant heart rate, what happens to cardiac output if venous return falls?** *1 mark*

Q **5(d). In cardiac failure, for a given heart rate and end-diastolic volume how does cardiac output compare to normal?** *1 mark*

Q **5(e). What happens to stroke volume if an increase in preload gives very high end-diastolic volumes?** *1 mark*

Q 5(f). In heart failure there is a downward shift of the ventricular performance curve. The reduced stroke volume results in incomplete chamber emptying during contraction. If in heart failure a weak ventricular systole gives incomplete chamber emptying, what will be the effect on the following ventricular systole?   *1 mark*

Q 6. What is an inotrope and what is a chronotrope?   *2 marks*

Q 7. Give an example of a positive inotrope and a positive chronotrope.

2 marks

Various pathophysiological changes occur in heart failure to compensate for the inability of the heart to pump sufficient blood to satisfy the needs of the body. Two of these are (a) salt and water retention and (b) stimulation of the sympathetic nervous system.

Salt and water retention is mediated by (a) the renin–angiotensin–aldosterone system and by (b) antidiuretic hormone.

Q 8. On which renal tubule cells do these two systems principally act? *2 marks*

	Tubules acted upon
Renin–angiotensin–aldosterone system	
Antidiuretic hormone	

Q 9. Which receptors, by reduced stimulation, activate the sympathetic nervous system when there is a fall in systolic blood pressure? *1 mark*

You reconsider the use of diuretics to address Mr Mayor's salt and water retention. You are familiar with bendroflumethiazide, furosemide and spironolactone.

Q 10. In the following table indicate the class of diuretic to which each of these drugs belongs and indicate which acts at sites A, B and C on the diagram (Figure 1.11). *3 marks*

	Class of diuretic
Bendroflumethiazide	
Furosemide	
Spironolactone	

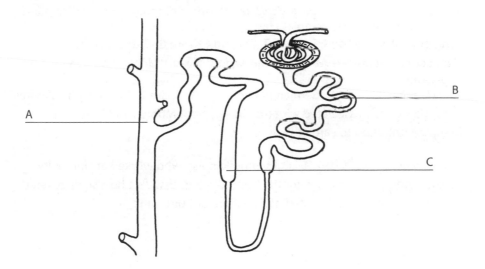

Figure 1.11: Site of drug action along the nephron.

CARDIOLOGY

(½ mark for each)

A –

B –

C –

You meet Mr Mayor in the canteen a couple of days later where he comes up to you to thank you. He mentions that he was very anxious during his admission and appreciated your support. You feel satisfied that you managed to diagnose and treat Mr Mayor effectively.

📖 BIBLIOGRAPHY

Guyton A C, Hall J E. 2006. *Textbook of Medical Physiology*, 11th edn. Philadelphia: Elsevier Saunders.

Kumar P, Clark M. 2005. *Clinical Medicine*, 6th edn. Edinburgh: Elsevier Saunders.

Longmore M, Wilkinson I, Turmeizi T, Cheung CK, Smith E. 2007. *Oxford Handbook of Clinical Medicine*, 7th edn. Oxford: Oxford University Press.

[a]Otto Frank (1865–1944), German physiologist. He spent a short time in Glasgow but is particularly associated with the University of Munich and is remembered for his contribution to cardiac physiology.

[b]Ernest Starling (1866–1927), English physiologist, who worked at University College London. He is noted for the Frank–Starling Law, but he also discovered secretin and described the Starling Equation for fluid shifts.

CARDIOLOGY
6. VENOUS CONDITIONS OF THE LOWER LIMB

Miss McGuire, a 58-year-old woman, presents to you, her GP. Her complaint is varicose veins in both legs. She is having aching pains in both lower limbs but especially on her right side, the worse of the two. Her shop job entails being on her feet a lot and the ache is proving troublesome. She has tried wearing elasticated stockings and, while they helped for a while, the pain is becoming troublesome again.

Q 1. Where do the long (great) and short (small) saphenous veins lie in relation to (a) the ankle joint and (b) the knee joint.   *4 marks*

Q 2. In which veins do the two saphenous veins terminate?   *2 marks*

On examination of Miss McGuire's legs, the long saphenous vein on both sides and other nearby superficial veins are seen to be varicose. There is brown discoloration of the skin of the medial calf on the right limb. On the right leg, just above the medial malleolus and at the mid-point of the medial calf, the varicosities are particularly obvious and are forming raised nodules.

Q 3. What is the likely explanation for the two sites of marked varicosity?

1½ marks

You also check for a saphena varix.

Q 4. Where is the 'saphenous opening'?

1 mark

Q 5. What is a saphena varix?

1 mark

Q 6. Which muscle in the lower limb is particularly important in the return of venous blood from the lower limb and why is this?

3 marks

Q 7. Indicate which of the following groups of veins have valves.

1½ marks

Veins	Yes or No
Superficial	
Deep	
Perforating	

Q 8. What are venae comitantes? *2 marks*

_____

_____

In view of the pain and also the clinical appearance, you decide to refer Miss McGuire to the local hospital for surgical management of her varicose veins.

Later the same morning a second patient presents with venous problems in the lower limb. Mrs Campbell, a 54-year-old woman, comes in complaining of a 2-day history of acute onset of pain in her left calf. She is struggling to walk because of the pain. On further questioning you discover she returned from a shopping trip to New York one week ago. Examination reveals a tender, erythematous, swollen left calf and a normal right calf.

Mrs Campbell is referred to the local hospital for further investigation. A Doppler[a] ultrasound reveals a deep venous thrombosis (DVT).

Q 9. Using the terms below, fill in the boxes of the coagulation cascade (Figure 1.12). *4 marks*

Activated factor X

Activated factor XIII

Fibrinogen

Hard fibrin

Prothrombin

Prothrombinase

Soft fibrin

Thrombin

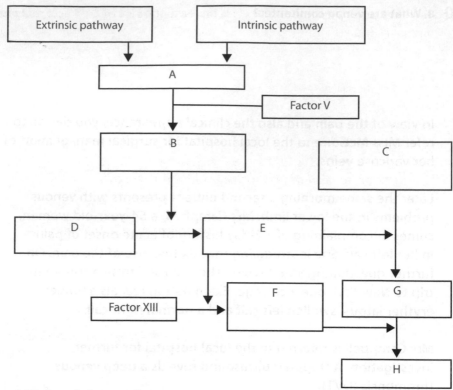

Figure 1.12: Coagulation cascade.

½ mark per box:

A –

B –

C –

D –

E –

F –

G –

H –

Q 10. What three physiological factors increase the risk of DVT according to Virchow's triad[b]? *3 marks*

It is decided to commence anticoagulation therapy.

Q 11. What potentially life-threatening complication of a DVT does anticoagulation aim to prevent? *1 mark*

Q 12. Choose three of the following agents and describe their mechanism of action: heparin, warfarin, aspirin and clopidogrel. *6 marks*

CARDIOLOGY

 BIBLIOGRAPHY

Ellis H. 2002. *Clinical Anatomy*, 10th edn. Oxford: Blackwell Publishing.

Kumar P, Clark M. 2005. *Clinical Medicine*, 6th edn. Edinburgh: Elsevier Saunders.

Sinnatamby C S. 1999. *Last's Anatomy: Regional and Applied*, 10th edn. Edinburgh: Churchill Livingstone.

[a]See Neurology Case 1.

[b]Rudolf Ludwig Karl Virchow (1821–1902), German doctor who made a number of medical discoveries including Virchow's node, an enlarged supraclavicular node indicative of upper gastrointestinal malignancy, and Virchow's triad, factors predisposing to deep venous thrombosis.

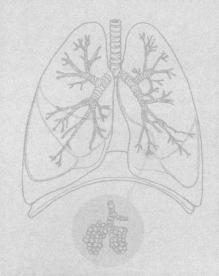

RESPIRATORY CASES: QUESTIONS

RESPIRATORY
1. CYSTIC FIBROSIS

You are a final year medical student with the on-call house officer in Accident and Emergency and are asked to see a breathless young girl with a cough. You are surprised to learn that Lucy is 14 years old. She appears much smaller. Her mother tells you that she has cystic fibrosis. You feel alarm, but not panic, as you have yet to study this. You remember that consideration of basic science is important in understanding any clinical problem.

Cystic fibrosis affects a number of organs including the lungs. Lucy's mother says that she is worried Lucy has developed 'yet another chest infection' since starting a social support group with other children affected by cystic fibrosis.

Q **1. Label the diagram of the lungs below (Figure 2.1).**   *6 marks*

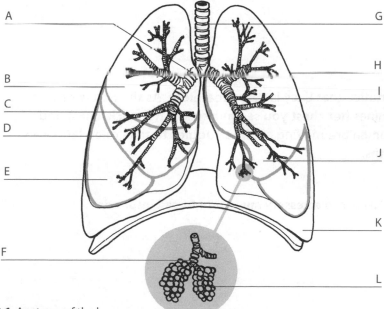

Figure 2.1: Anatomy of the lung.

½ mark for each of the following:

A –

B –

C –

D –

E –

F –

G –

H –

I –

J –

K –

L –

You notice that Lucy is very breathless. As the house officer examines her chest you see muscles of her neck, chest and abdomen are moving as she struggles to take deep laboured breaths.

Q 2(a). Name *two* accessory muscles of forced inspiration.   *2 marks*

Q 2(b). Name *four* **accessory muscles of forced expiration.** *2 marks*

As you watch, Lucy gives a cough. As this happens, the lateral edge of a muscle becomes prominent on each side of her chest. The muscle edge is seen to run from the lower back to the humerus and to squeeze the chest as Lucy coughs.

Q 3. Which muscle is this and what is its nerve supply? *1 mark*

Lucy has been coughing up copious sputum and a sample is collected for microbiological analysis. The house officer tells you that normal respiratory epithelial secretions contain a large number of chemo-protective agents such as lactoferrin and defensins. These help to prevent respiratory infections in healthy individuals.

Q 4. Name *two* **normal respiratory epithelial chemo-protective secretions (in addition to the two examples above).** *1 mark*

Q 5. Name *two* **cells of the innate immune system that you might expect to be present in Lucy's lung at this time.** *2 marks*

Infection seems likely and the house officer orders a chest x-ray. You anticipate being required to interpret the plain film and consider the relevant anatomy.

Here is the radiograph. It shows changes in the right upper lobe and consolidation in the middle part of the left lung field.

Q **6. Some normal anatomical features have been labelled. Please identify A–H.** *4 marks*

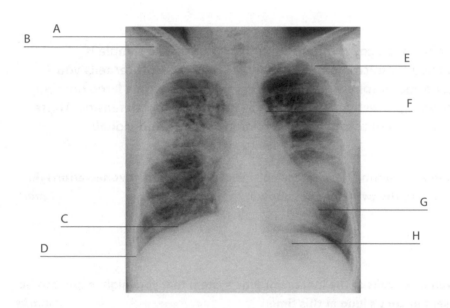

Figure 2.2: Lucy's chest radiograph.

A –

B –

C –

D –

E –

F –

G –

H –

Meanwhile, Lucy's brother, 2-year-old Tom, is running riot around the Accident and Emergency Department. You wonder if he is also affected by cystic fibrosis. The doctor takes a family history and asks you to sketch a family tree into Lucy's case notes.

Q 7. Using the family history notes below, draw a family tree indicating:

a. Lucy has cystic fibrosis.

b. Tom does not appear to have cystic fibrosis. (His 'Guthrie test' was negative. He has yet to have DNA analysis testing for cystic fibrosis genes.)

c. Their parents are both in good health.

d. Lucy's mother is expecting a third child, genotype unknown.

e. Lucy's maternal grandparents are both alive and well.

f. Lucy's uncle (mother's brother) died from cystic fibrosis, aged 24. *4 marks*

Q 8. What is the Guthrie Test?   *2 marks*

_____

_____

Q 9. State the mode of inheritance of cystic fibrosis.   *1 mark*

_____

Q **10. State the chance that Tom is a carrier for the gene mutation which causes cystic fibrosis.** *1 mark*

Q **11. State the chance that the unborn sibling will have cystic fibrosis.** *1 mark*

Q **12. Define the term gene.** *1 mark*

Q **13. What is the name of the protein affected by the gene defect, associated with cystic fibrosis?** *1 mark*

Q **14. Name the two ions affected by the defective protein in cystic fibrosis.** *1 mark*

Lucy is admitted to the ward and started on intravenous antibiotics. You are pleased to see an improvement in her respiratory infection over the following few days.

📖 BIBLIOGRAPHY

Boon N A, Colledge N R, Walker B R, Hunter J A A. 2006. *Davidson's Principles and Practices of Medicine*, 20th edn. Edinburgh: Elsevier Churchill Livingstone.

Hodson M, Geddes D, Bush A. 2007. *Cystic Fibrosis*, 3rd edn. London: Hodder Arnold.

RESPIRATORY

2. TUBERCULOSIS

You are a locum GP in a busy practice in the middle of a morning surgery, when you are phoned by an anxious woman. Her father, 72-year-old Mr Stevens, has been quite unwell for over 2 weeks, and does not seem to be improving. He has a cough and a spit which is green at the moment and occasionally blood-stained. Recently, he has also been complaining of night sweats. Mr Stevens is reluctant to come and see you. He has a history of chronic obstructive pulmonary disease and suffers chest infections fairly regularly. He has told his daughter his chest has seemed worse in the past few months.

Q 1. Suggest four possible differential diagnoses. *2 marks*

After the discussion with his daughter you decide you should probably visit Mr Stevens. On your way over in the car you begin thinking about the anatomy and histology of the respiratory system.

Q 2. Identify A–C in this diagram of the end of a bronchiole (Figure 2.5).

3 marks

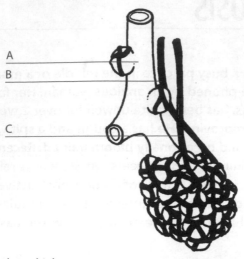

Figure 2.5: The bronchiole.

One for each of the following:

A –

B –

C –

Q 3. Name the two main cell types found in the wall of an alveolus and describe their functions. *2 marks*

Q 4. At which stage of life are babies theoretically capable of respiratory survival because these cells begin functioning? *1 mark*

You arrive at Mr Stevens's house to find him in bed, coughing, and very hot and clammy. He is coherent and you take a brief history from him. You discover he has been feeling like this for over 2 weeks, and has had frequent chest infections in the last year for which he has received antibiotics. He has a history of chronic obstructive pulmonary disease, hypertension and diabetes. He uses a fluticasone and salmeterol inhaler, and takes ramipril, aspirin and metformin. He has a vague memory of his grandfather having similar symptoms when he was a boy, but assumed it was because he was always smoking. Mr Stevens stopped smoking 5 years ago but smoked 30 cigarettes a day before that when he worked in the shipyard. He still enjoys a few whiskies.

Q 5. What is the rationale of the fluticasone and salmeterol in the inhaler? **2 marks**

Q 6. Why is Mr Stevens taking ramipril and metformin and what types of drug are they? **2 marks**

On examination you find reduced bilateral air entry, reduced chest expansion, crackles in both bases and a small area of dullness over the right base.

Q 7. List four causes of a dull percussion note. **2 marks**

You suspect Mr Stevens may have tuberculosis (TB) and he is admitted to hospital.

Q 8. Name the most likely causative organism.   *1 mark*

Q 9. Describe this organism   *4 marks*

Coccus or rod?	
Aerobe or anaerobe?	
Gram positive or Gram negative?	
Produces spores/does not produce spores?	

Q 10. What is the Ziehl-Neelsen stain?   *2 marks*

Mr Stevens is diagnosed as having pulmonary tuberculosis.

The consultant takes a group of students to see Mr Stevens. He asks them where they think he got tuberculosis. Since the patient is not aware of any TB contacts, they suggest secondary infection from someone that may not have been noticeably unwell, or reactivation due to his lowered immune status (COPD and diabetes). The consultant asks the students to think about primary TB infection in childhood.

Q 11. What name is given to the site of primary infection in the lungs? *1 mark*

Q 12. **What is miliary tuberculosis?** *1 mark*

Q 13. **Name the type of immune response that occurs against tubercle bacilli.** *1 mark*

Q 14. **What part of the organism triggers this reaction?** *1 mark*

Below is a diagram of a chronic granuloma, typically associated with tuberculosis. It consists of a central necrotic core, surrounded by three cellular layers.

Q 15. **The layers are labelled A–C. What is the general cellular content of each layer?** *3 marks*

A –

B –

C –

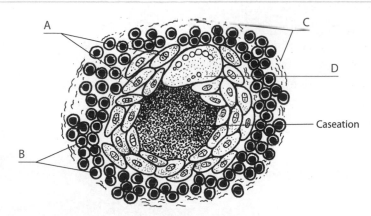

Figure 2.6: Chronic granuloma.

Q 16. A large cell is labelled D. What type is it? *1 mark*

The students begin thinking about the fact that the body develops immunity to certain microbes and how science has used this to produce vaccines.

Q 17. Name the pre-vaccination test and the vaccination for tuberculosis. *1 mark*

📖 BIBLIOGRAPHY

McMinn R M H, Gaddum-Rosse P, Hutchings R T, Logan B M. 1995. *Functional and Clinical Anatomy*. London: Mosby.

Reid R, Roberts F. 2005. *Pathology Illustrated*, 6th edn. Edinburgh: Churchill Livingstone.

Woolfe N, Wotherspoon A C, Young M. 2002. *Essentials of Pathology*. Edinburgh: W. B. Saunders.

RESPIRATORY

RESPIRATORY
3. RESPIRATORY TRACT INFECTION

You are on duty in general practice one afternoon for urgent house calls when you are asked by the receptionist to visit 75-year-old Mr Gray, a widower living alone and normally very self-sufficient. His daughter, who lives about 50 miles away, has phoned the practice to say that she is very worried. Her father had had a bad cold and sore throat for a few days. Today he had sounded so strange on the telephone that she had driven over immediately. She had found her father to be confused, breathless, coughing and 'burning up'.

Q 1. Give the two most likely diagnoses to account for this presentation.

2 marks

You find Mr Gray, a thin man of moderate height, lying propped up in bed. He has a greyish, anxious appearance with a blue tinge to his lips and is difficult to rouse. Blood pressure is 110/70 mmHg, with a regular pulse rate of 108 beats per minute. His temperature is 40.5ºC. Mr Gray has an increased respiratory rate and is using accessory muscles of respiration.

Q 2. What is the normal respiratory rate?

1 mark

Q 3. Which muscle is normally responsible for *quiet* inspiration?

1 mark

Q 4. What mechanism brings about quiet expiration?   *1 mark*

Q 5. What are the main 'accessory muscles of respiration'?   *2 marks*

Palpation revealed decreased expansion on the left side of the
chest and increased vocal fremitus over the left base. Percussion
revealed dullness over the left base.

Q 6. What is meant by the 'left lung base'?   *1 mark*

Q 7. Where does the lung base lie with respect to the surface anatomy of the
chest wall?   *1 mark*

Auscultation revealed bronchial breathing over the lower part of
the left side of the chest along with generalised bilateral coarse
crepitations and rhonchi. There was increased vocal resonance on
the lower left side of the chest.

Q 8. What does increased vocal resonance indicate?   *1 mark*

Q 9. Identify A–F on the following radiograph (Figure 2.7).   *3 marks*

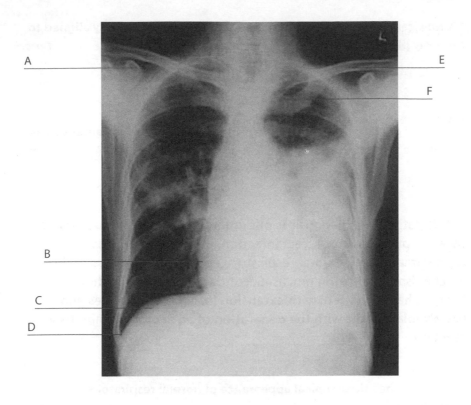

Figure 2.7: Chest radiograph.

A –

B –

C –

D –

E –

F –

Q 10. How can you tell that the patient's chest has been properly aligned to the x-ray plate?   *1 mark*

Q 11. Why, if possible, is a chest radiograph taken as a postero-anterior view, ie with the front of the patient's chest against the X-ray plate?   *1 mark*

In this patient the diagnosis is pneumonia. It is usually precipitated by an upper respiratory tract infection, probably viral. This will have damaged the normal respiratory epithelium with loss of the mechanism for clearing mucus. Secondary bacterial infection is likely to have followed, with extension into the bronchioles and the alveolar spaces with the generation of an acute inflammatory reaction.

Q 12. What is the microscopical appearance of normal respiratory epithelium?   *2 marks*

Q 13. Where does mucus in the respiratory tract come from?   *1 mark*

Q 14. What is the normal mechanism for clearing the mucus?   *1 mark*

Q 15. As a result of the bacterial infection, what type of leukocyte is likely to invade the alveolar spaces? *1 mark*

The host defences, which normally protect the lungs from infection, have obviously been overcome.

Q 16. List any four of these non-specific (innate) antimicrobial defence mechanisms in the respiratory tract. *2 marks*

Because Mr Gray is living alone, is somewhat confused and has severe breathlessness and cyanosis, you arrange for him to be admitted to hospital. On admission arterial blood gases are checked on air. The results were as follows:

	$[H^+]$ (nmol/l)	$PaCO_2$ (kPa)	HCO_3 (mmol/l)	PaO_2 (kPa)	SaO_2 (%)
Reference range	36–44	4.6–6.0	22–28	10.5–13.5	>95
Mr Gray	61	4.0	11.8	6.8	79

Q 17. Explain these arterial blood gas findings on air. *3 marks*

Q 18. Where are the two main sites of peripheral chemoreceptors? *1 mark*

Q 19. Which nerve(s) innervate these chemoreceptors? *1 mark*

Q 20. Describe the anatomical pathway of an oxygen molecule in a healthy lung as it diffuses from the alveolar gas to the haemoglobin molecule across the *thinnest* part of the blood air barrier. *2 marks*

Q 21. Are lung capillaries fenestrated? *1 mark*

📖 BIBLIOGRAPHY

Ganong W F. 2005. *Review of Medical Physiology*, 22nd edn. New York: McGraw-Hill Medical.

RESPIRATORY
4. ASTHMA

You are a house officer working in the acute receiving ward when Mr Roxburgh, a 35-year-old, is admitted with sudden onset of severe left-sided chest pain and increasing shortness of breath. He is breathless with central cyanosis. Examination of the thorax shows decreased expansion on the left side which is hyper-resonant to percussion. The trachea is deviated to the right and the apex beat is palpable in the 5th intercostal space 1 cm from the left sternal edge.

His chest X-ray on admission is shown below

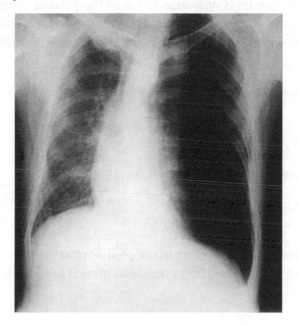

Q 1. What is the immediate cause of his acute symptoms?   *2 marks*

His systolic blood pressure is 100 mmHg.

Q 2. What might this measurement indicate?   *1 mark*

Q 3. The radiograph shows that the mediastinum has shifted. What two findings on the clinical examination also suggest that this has occurred?   *2 marks*

A wide-bore needle is now inserted into the pleural cavity via the 6th intercostal space in the mid-axillary line and air allowed to escape under pressure. Mr Roxburgh begins to feel much easier.

Q 4. What is the pleural cavity?   *1 mark*

Q 5. What is the costodiaphragmatic recess?   *1 mark*

Q 6. In Mr Roxburgh, the pressure in the pleural cavity had risen. Which of the following is the most likely mean intrapleural pressure in a normal subject?   *1 mark*

A: −6 cmH$_2$O

B: 0 cmH$_2$O

C: 10 cmH$_2$O

D: 760 cmH$_2$O

As well as breathlessness, Mr Roxburgh complains of pleuritic-type chest pain.

Q 7. From which particular tissue layer is the pain arising? *1 mark*

After air had been allowed out of the pleural cavity, a water seal drain, inserted as before, replaced the needle.

Q 8. Name four muscles that the drain will penetrate. *2 marks*

Q 9. Other than the muscles, what structures are at risk in: (a) the upper part of the intercostal space and (b) the lower part of the intercostal space? *2 marks*

You now discover that Mr Roxburgh is an asthmatic and had had an exacerbation of this the day before he became acutely breathless.

After he has recovered from his acute asthma and from his pneumothorax he has respiratory function tests carried out.

Q 10. On the following diagram of lung volumes (Figure 2.8), which functional parameters are represented by labels I, II and III? *3 marks*

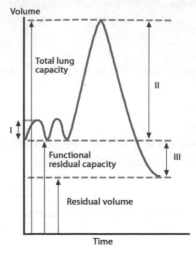

Figure 2.8: Lung volumes.

1 mark for each of the following:	**II –**
I –	**III –**

Q **11. How is total lung capacity defined?** *1 mark*

Q **12. Approximately what is the normal total lung capacity in a male adult?** *1 mark*

A report comes back from the Pulmonary Function Laboratory with the values shown in the table below.

Lung volumes	Normal ref range	Patient	Patient after bronchodilator
FEV 1 (litres)	4.0	2.3	3.5
FVC (litres)	5.0	4.1	4.8
FEV/FVC	80%	56%	73%

Q 13. Define the terms FEV and FVC as used here.　　　　*2 marks*

Q 14. Explain the findings.　　　　*3 marks*

Q 15. To which of the following levels of the respiratory tract do smooth muscle fibres extend?　　　　*1 mark*

Portion of airway	Smooth muscle present?
Lobar bronchi	
Segmental bronchi	
Terminal bronchioles	
Respiratory bronchioles	
Alveolar walls	

Q 16. How are the smooth muscle fibres orientated in the smaller airways?　　　　*1 mark*

Q 17. In asthma, name two of the major cell types responsible for the release of chemical mediators that cause bronchial smooth muscle to contract.　　　　*1 mark*

69

Mr Roxburgh has a history consistent with atopic asthma.

Q **18. What type of hypersensitivity response is this?**   *1 mark*

Prior to this episode Mr Roxburgh used regular inhaled salbutamol to control his asthma symptoms.

Q **19. What is the mode of action of this drug?**   *1 mark*

During this episode he required oral steroids as well and it is decided to discharge him on a combination treatment, 'Symbicort' – budesonide and formoterol fumarate.

Q **20. What is the mode of action of each of these?**   *2 marks*

📖 BIBLIOGRAPHY

Ganong W F. 2005. *Review of Medical Physiology*, 22nd edn. New York: McGraw-Hill Medical.

Kumar P, Clark M. 2005. *Clinical Medicine*, 6th edn. Edinburgh: Elsevier Saunders.

West J B. 2001. *Pulmonary Physiology and Pathophysiology: An Integrated Case-Based Approach*. Philadelphia: Lippincott, Williams and Wilkins.

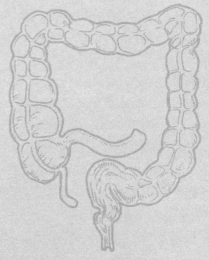

GASTROENTEROLOGY CASES:
QUESTIONS

GASTROENTEROLOGY
1. EPIGASTRIC PAIN

Mrs Jones, a 43-year-old woman, has been admitted to the Accident and Emergency Department with sudden onset of severe pain in the epigastric region which radiated through to her back. She complains of feeling nauseous and has vomited twice. On examination, she is pale and her sclerae are jaundiced. She is tachycardic with a pulse rate of 110 beats per minute. Her blood pressure is 90/60 mmHg. Abdominal examination reveals ecchymosis of the flanks, tenderness in the epigastric area and bowel sounds are present. You suspect acute pancreatitis.

Q 1. Label this diagram of structures in the upper abdomen (Figure 3.1).

3 marks

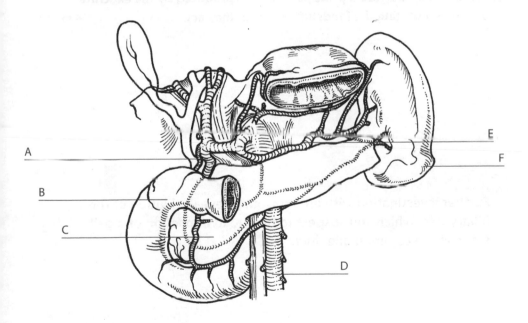

Figure 3.1: Anatomy of the upper abdomen.

½ **mark per correct label (3 marks in total):**

A – _____

B – _____

C – _____

D – _____

E – _____

F – _____

Blood tests reveal high serum amylase levels and raised blood glucose, supporting your suspicions of acute pancreatitis.

Q **2. Name four individual principal enzymes produced by the exocrine pancreas and state the foodstuff on which they act.**   *4 marks*

_____

_____

_____

_____

Further investigation with an ultrasound reveals dilation of the biliary tree, which you suspect to be due to impaction of a gall stone in the common bile duct.

Q 3. **Label this diagram of the biliary tree (Figure 3.2).**   *4 marks*

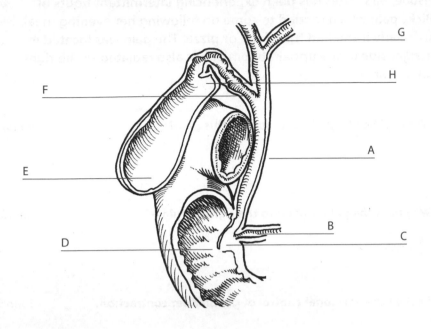

Figure 3.2: The biliary tree.

½ mark for each correct label, 4 marks in total:

A –

B –

C –

D –

E –

F –

G –

H –

On further questioning it is revealed that, prior to the present episode, Mrs Jones has been experiencing intermittent bouts of colicky pain which tended to come on following her evening meal, particularly if she had fried food or pizza. The pain was located in the right side of the upper abdomen but also radiated to the right shoulder area.

Q 4. What is the likely clinical cause of this pain?   *1 mark*

Q 5. Why does the pain radiate to the right shoulder?   *2 marks*

Q 6. Explain the hormonal control of gallbladder contraction.   *1 mark*

Along with the amylase and glucose results the following results of liver function tests are received.

Blood results:

Test	Alkaline phosphatase	Alanine transaminase	Bilirubin	Conjugated bilirubin
Result	1832 U/l (39–117 U/l)	186 U/l (5–40 U/l)	204 µmol/l (< 17 µmol/l)	166 µmol/l

Q 7. The biochemistry results indicate that Mrs Jones has obstructive (post-hepatic) jaundice. Explain the reasoning that leads to this diagnosis.

3 marks

Q 8. Bilirubin is formed from haem during the destruction of old or damaged erythrocytes in the spleen. Please answer the following questions on bilirubin metabolism after it leaves the spleen. Each question is worth ½ mark. *4 marks*

Q 8(a). Is the bilirubin produced by the spleen soluble in water? *½ mark*

Q 8(b). To which substance is bilirubin bound as it is passed in the venous blood from the spleen to the liver? *½ mark*

Q 8(c). By which two veins does the bound bilirubin pass from the spleen to the liver? *½ mark for both veins*

Q 8(d). Which cell organelle is responsible for conjugation of bilirubin? *½ mark*

Q 8(e). Into which lumen is conjugated bilirubin directly secreted by hepatocytes? *½ mark*

Q 8(f). What is the source of the enzymes that reduce bilirubin to urobilinogen in the bowel? *½ mark*

GASTROENTEROLOGY

Q 8(g). Which vein carries resorbed urobilinogen from the terminal ileum to the portal vein?   ½ mark

Q 8(h). As well as loss in the stools, by what other means is urobilinogen lost from the body?   ½ mark

Having presented with jaundice, Mrs Jones underwent urgent endoscopic retrograde cholangiopancreatography (ERCP). This confirmed the presence of a gallstone impacted in the common bile duct, which was subsequently removed. The stone was mainly composed of cholesterol.

Q 9. Give two functions of cholesterol?   2 marks

During her admission Mrs Jones had a CT scan with contrast to exclude pancreatic necrosis or abscess formation. Below is a CT scan of a normal upper abdomen.

Q **10. Identify structures A–H (Figure 3.3).** *4 marks*

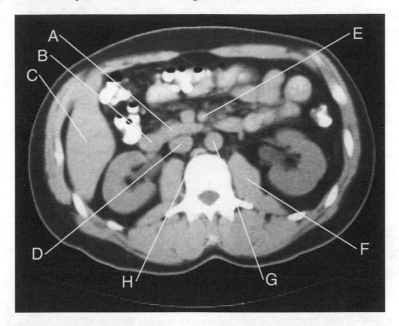

Figure 3.3: CT of abdomen.

4 marks total – ½ mark each:

A –

B –

C –

D –

E –

F –

G –

H –

Mrs Jones was managed conservatively with fluids, analgesia and her hyperglycaemia was corrected using insulin. Before discharge she is started on a statin.

Q 11. Explain how statins work. *2 marks*

📖 BIBLIOGRAPHY

Boon N A, Colledge N R, Walker B R, Hunter J A A. 2006. *Davidson's Principles and Practices of Medicine*, 20th edn. Edinburgh: Elsevier Churchill Livingstone.

Burkitt H G, Quick C R G. 2002. *Essential Surgery: Problems, Diagnosis and Management*. Edinburgh: Churchill Livingstone.

Garden O, Bradbury A, Forsythe J. 2002. *Principles and Practice of Surgery*, 4th edn. Edinburgh: Elsevier.

Kumar P, Clark M. 2005. *Clinical Medicine*, 6th edn. Edinburgh: Elsevier Saunders.

Pocock G, Richards C. 2004. Human Physiology: The Basis of Medicine, 2nd edn. Oxford Core Texts.

GASTROENTEROLOGY

GASTROENTEROLOGY
2. INFLAMMATORY BOWEL DISEASE

Mr McDonald, a 29-year-old plumber, presents to his GP with a 2-week history of bloody diarrhoea and abdominal pain. He has been feeling generally unwell but has not experienced vomiting. On further questioning he tells his GP he has been passing stools 5–6 times per day and has also been passing mucus. Mr McDonald has not lost any weight recently but his appetite has been reduced. At this stage, two main differential diagnoses are considered, inflammatory bowel disease (IBD) and infection. There was no history of overseas travel.

On initial examination, there is mild peri-umbilical tenderness and blood and mucus are identified on rectal examination. A stool sample is collected and sent for microbiological analysis.

Q 1. **Name four organisms which commonly cause bloody diarrhoea.** *2 marks*

Stool sample results are negative and Mr McDonald continues to suffer from bloody diarrhoea. Routine blood tests are taken at initial presentation including full blood count, urea and electrolytes and C-reactive protein (CRP).

The results are as follows:

	Mr McDonald's results	Normal range
Hb	10.3 g/dl	12.5–16.5 g/dl
MCV	88 fl	83–101 fl
WCC	$12.2 \times 10^9 \, l^{-1}$	$(4.0–11.0) \times 10^9 \, l^{-1}$
Platelets	$296 \times 10^9 \, l^{-1}$	$(150–400) \times 10^9 \, l^{-1}$
CRP	64 mg/l	< 10 mg/l

A blood film is also examined and the erythrocytes appear normal.

Q 2(a). Where is CRP produced? *1 mark*

Q 2(b). What is the clinical significance of elevated CRP? *1 mark*

Q 3. What type of anaemia is this? *1 mark*

Due to the presence of anaemia, tests of serum ferritin, folate, B_{12} and iron are requested. B_{12}, folate and iron are found to be low and ferritin levels are raised. When body iron stores are low, ferritin production is usually down-regulated.

Q 4(a). Why is the ferritin level elevated in this patient? *1 mark*

Q 4(b). What ionic form of iron is most commonly ingested, ferric or ferrous? *1 mark*

Q 4(c). What ionic form of iron is absorbed in the GI tract? *1 mark*

GASTROENTEROLOGY

Q 4(d). Where in the gastrointestinal tract does iron absorption occur? *1 mark*

Q 4(e). How is iron transported into cells and what is its fate after this? *4 marks*

A colonoscopy is arranged for Mr McDonald.

Q 5(a). List the four main histological layers of the colon. *2 marks*

Q 5(b). The longitudinal muscle fibres of the muscularis externa of the colon are arranged into three bands in the colon. What are these called? *1 mark*

Q 5(c). Between which layers would you find the myenteric plexus (Auerbach's plexus)? *1 mark*

Biopsies of the colon were taken and histology results are awaited.

Q 6(a). The colon is illustrated below (Figure 3.4). Label the diagram. *4 marks*

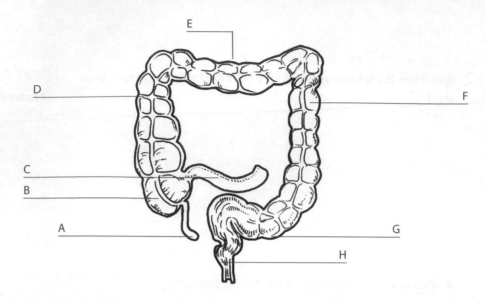

Figure 3.4: Diagram of colon.

½ mark for each of the following:

A –

B –

C –

D –

E –

F –

G –

H –

GASTROENTEROLOGY

Q 6(b). List two of these structures that are retroperitoneal.   *1 mark*

Q 6(c). Name one other retroperitoneal structure.   *1 mark*

Q 6(d). What is the blood supply of the ascending colon?   *1 mark*

During colonoscopy, the macroscopic appearance is suggestive of inflammatory bowel disease (IBD) with diffuse bleeding and inflammation. The two main subgroups of IBD are ulcerative colitis and Crohn's disease.

Q 7. Complete the following table relating to pathological differences between ulcerative colitis and Crohn's disease.[a]   *5 marks*

	Crohn's disease	Ulcerative colitis
Part of GI tract affected		
Are the lesions continuous?		
Which layers of the gut wall are affected?		
How are goblet cell numbers affected?		
State one other common pathological appearance that is characteristic of the disease		

Mr McDonald is commenced on corticosteroids to control the initial episode of IBD. He remains well.

Q 8. Which colonic pathology can develop in patients who have long-standing, inflammatory bowel disease, particularly ulcerative colitis? *1 mark*

📖 BIBLIOGRAPHY

Ganong W F. 2005. *Review of Medical Physiology*, 22nd edn. New York: McGraw-Hill Medical.

Guyton A C, Hall J E. 2000. *Textbook of Medical Physiology*, 10th edn. Philadelphia: WB Saunders Co.

Kumar P, Clark M. 2005. *Clinical Medicine*, 6th edn. Edinburgh: Elsevier Saunders.

Kumar V, Cotran R, Robbins S. 2003. *Basic Pathology*, 7th edn. London: WB Saunders.

MacSween R N M, Whaley K. 1992. *Muir's Textbook of Pathology*, 13th edn. London: Arnold.

[a]Burrill Bernard Crohn (1884–1983), American gastroenterologist. Crohn's disease is named after him although it had been described independently in 1904 by Polish surgeon Antoni Lesniowski.

GASTROENTEROLOGY

GASTROENTEROLOGY
3. PAINLESS JAUNDICE

Mr McMurdo is a 57-year-old man who presents because he has become jaundiced. He has lost weight over the last few weeks and recently has been feeling tired and somewhat depressed. He had previously been in good health. On abdominal examination, there is no tenderness but the fundus of the gallbladder is palpable.

Q 1. What is the surface marking for the fundus of the gallbladder?   *1 mark*

Q 2. In surgery, what is Courvoisier's[a] Law?   *1 mark*

You also notice that Mr McMurdo has a number of scratch marks on his arms and legs. He volunteers that he has an itch which is extremely distressing and complains that it keeps him awake at night.

Q 3(a). Explain the likely cause of his itch.   *1 mark*

Q 3(b). Cholestyramine is used to treat this itch. Briefly outline its mechanism of action.   *1 mark*

87

Q 3(c). Name two other medications that might also help. *1 mark*

Blood tests indicate the presence of obstructive jaundice.

Tests are also carried out to investigate the synthetic function of Mr McMurdo's liver.

Q 4. Complete this table to indicate and explain the abnormal test result expected. *4 marks*

Test used	Abnormality expected	Brief explanation outlining why this would occur
Prothrombin time (PT)		
Albumin		

During the history, Mr McMurdo said he has lost 7 kg in weight over the past 6 months. More recently he has also noticed a change in his bowel habit. He complains of pale, whitish, greasy stools that are often difficult to flush away (steatorrhea).

Q 5. Explain why his stools are white. *1 mark*

Q 6. Name two substances formed from bile pigments that give the stools their characteristic colour. *2 marks*

Mr McMurdo also complains of darkened urine.

Q 7. What two biochemical abnormalities in the urine are seen in this type of jaundice? *2 marks*

Due to your clinical suspicions you refer Mr McMurdo urgently for endoscopic retrograde cholangiopancreatography (ERCP). At ERCP a protrusion was seen at the head of the pancreas and biopsy samples were taken.

Q 8. To which region of the peritoneal cavity is the pancreas particularly related? *1 mark*

Q 9. How is a pancreatic mass most likely to cause jaundice? *3 marks*

GASTROENTEROLOGY

Q **10. Label this diagram of the liver and biliary tree (Figure 3.5).**   *6 marks*

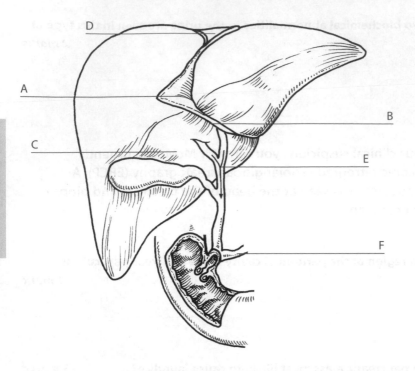

Figure 3.5: The liver and biliary tree.

A _____

B _____

C _____

D _____

E _____

F _____

Later in the day of his ERCP, Mr McMurdo started to complain of severe epigastric pain that radiated through to his back.

Q 11. What is the likely cause of this pain?   *1 mark*

Q 12. Explain Mr McMurdo's back pain.   *1 mark*

On examination Mr McMurdo has a bluish discoloration of his umbilicus and his flanks.

Q 13. Name these two clinical signs.   *1 mark*

As a result of this complication, Mr McMurdo is admitted to ITU and, fortunately, soon recovers from it. The histology from his biopsy samples returns, showing an adenocarcinoma of the pancreas. Further staging indicates that the tumour is resectable. The most common curative operation carried out for head of pancreas is a Whipple's procedure, which involves the en bloc excision of the distal two-thirds of the stomach, distal common bile duct, gallbladder, head of the pancreas and duodenum.

Due to the removal of such a large proportion of the pancreas, malabsorption is likely to occur.

Q 14. The pancreolauryl test can be used to assess exocrine pancreatic function. Briefly outline how this test works.   *3 marks*

91

📖 BIBLIOGRAPHY

Boon NA, Colledge NR, Walker BR, Hunter JAA. 2006. *Davidson's Principles and Practices of Medicine*, 20th edn. Edinburgh: Elsevier Churchill Livingstone.

Hempfling W, Dilger K, Beuers U. 2003. Systematic review: ursodeoxycholic acid – adverse effects and drug interactions. *Alimentary Pharmacology and Therapeutics*, **18**, 963–973.

Kumar P, Clark M. 2005. *Clinical Medicine*, 6th edn. Edinburgh: Elsevier Saunders.

Provan D, Krentz A. 2002. *Oxford Handbook of Clinical and Laboratory Investigation*. Oxford: Oxford University Press.

Smith ME, Morton DG. 2001. *The Digestive System*. Edinburgh: Churchill Livingstone.

Twycross R, Greaves MW, Handwerker H, Jones EA, Libretto SE, Szepietowski JC, Zylicz Z. 2003. Itch: scratching more than the surface. *Quarterly Journal of Medicine*, **96**, 7–23.

[a]Ludwig Courvoisier (1843–1918), Swiss surgeon who became Professor of Surgery at the University of Basle. Courvoisier's Law was first stated in a book published by him in 1890 on the pathology and surgery of the gall bladder.

GASTROENTEROLOGY
4. LIVER DISEASE

Mr Fraser is a 56-year-old man who presents to his GP with a 4-day history of worsening yellow discoloration of his skin and eyes. He is thin, has lost his appetite and complains of nausea, tiredness and upper abdominal discomfort especially on the right side. On examination he is markedly jaundiced and you find that he has an enlarged liver, ascites and gynaecomastia, but no spleen is palpable.

Q 1. Define ascites. *1 mark*

Q 2. Give three conditions that might give rise to ascites. *1½ marks*

Q 3. Explain the pathophysiology of gynaecomastia. *2 marks*

Q 4. In the presence of portal hypertension the spleen may be enlarged. Why is this? *1 mark*

Q 5. Supply the missing words.   *2 marks*

2 marks in total: ½ mark for each:

The normal spleen lies in the left _____ region of the abdomen. The spleen lies at the level of the ____ to the 11th ribs. A normal spleen lies posterior to the mid-axillary line and is separated from the left lung by the _____ covered superiorly by the _____ and inferiorly by the peritoneum.

As you examine Mr Fraser further, you begin to think about the histological structure of the liver.

Q 6. In the diagram below (Figure 3.6) identify unit of liver A and unit of liver structure B. Identify features C, D and E.   *5 marks*

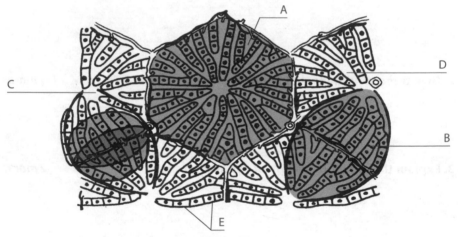

Figure 3.6: Histological structure of the liver.

A –

B –

C –

D –

E –

GASTROENTEROLOGY

Q 7. Where are the portal tracts situated? *1 mark*

Q 8. Name the three tubular structures found in a portal tract. *1 mark*

Q 9. Give two ways in which the cellular lining of the liver sinusoids is specialised to aid liver function. *2 marks*

Q 10. What is the perisinusoidal space (of Disse) and what function does it assist? *1 mark*

Upon further questioning Mr Fraser tells you that he is an alcoholic with a prolonged history of excess drinking over about ten years. He has been drinking about 40 units a week with recent binges. You suspect alcoholic liver disease.

Q 11(a). What substance is produced in the first step of alcohol metabolism catalysed by cytoplasmic alcohol dehydrogenase? *1 mark*

Q 11(b). Is this metabolic pathway inducible? *1 mark*

Q 11(c). Which other metabolic pathway is involved in alcohol metabolism? *1 mark*

Blood results:

Test	γGT (IU/l)	Alkaline phosphatase (U/l)	AST (IU/l)	ALT (IU/l)	Total bilirubin (µmol/l)
Result	148 (11–58)	136 (39–117)	151 (12–40)	72 (5–40)	130 (less than 17)

Q 12(a). Define the type of jaundice. *1 mark*

Q 12(b). What is the significance of each of the following observations:

Q i. Markedly raised levels of aspartate transaminase and alanine transaminase? *½ mark*

Q ii. Markedly elevated gamma-glutamyl transferase? *½ mark*

Q iii. Elevated level of alkaline phosphatase? *½ mark*

A full blood count has also been carried out and a macrocytic anaemia with a neurophilia is reported.

Q 13. What are the two most likely explanations for the macrocytosis? *1 mark*

Q 14. Put the following features of alcoholic liver disease in order of most likely progression. *1 mark*

Alcoholic hepatitis

Cirrhosis

Hepatocellular carcinoma

Steatosis (fatty liver)

A liver biopsy is carried out on Mr Fraser. It confirms your clinical suspicion that he has alcoholic hepatitis.

Q 15. Give four characteristic features of alcoholic hepatitis as seen on light microscopy of the biopsy specimen. *4 marks*

The biopsy and radiological imaging suggest that Mr Fraser's liver disease has not progressed to cirrhosis.

Q 16. Define cirrhosis. *1 mark*

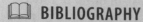 **BIBLIOGRAPHY**

Boon N A, Colledge N R, Walker B R, Hunter J A A. 2006. *Davidson's Principles and Practice of Medicine*, 20th edn. Edinburgh: Elsevier Churchill Livingstone.

Fawcett D W. 1994. *A Textbook of Histology*. New York: Chapman and Hall.

Kumar P, Clark M. 2005. *Clinical Medicine*, 6th edn. Edinburgh: Elsevier Saunders.

McPhee S J, Ganong W F. 2006. *Pathophysiology of Disease*, 5th edn. New York: Lange Medical Books/McGraw-Hill.

Provan D, Krentz A. 2002. *Oxford Handbook of Clinical and Laboratory Investigation*. Oxford: Oxford University Press.

Smith M E, Morton D G. 2001. *The Digestive System*. Edinburgh: Churchill Livingstone.

Sorbi D, Boynton J, Lindor K D. 1999. The ratio of aspartate aminotransferase to alanine aminotransferase: potential value in differentiating nonalcoholic steatohepatitis from alcoholic liver disease. *Am J Gastroenterol*, **94**, 1018–1022.

GASTROENTEROLOGY

GASTROENTEROLOGY
5. GASTRO-OESOPHAGEAL REFLUX DISEASE

Mr Anderson is a 57-year-old businessman who smokes 15 cigarettes per day and typically has his main meal in the later evening along with a glass of wine. He presents to his GP with heartburn, belching and waterbrash. His GP suspects that he is suffering from gastro-oesophageal reflux disease.

Q 1. Where does the pharynx become continuous with the oesophagus?

1 mark

Q 2. In which regions of the mediastinum does the oesophagus lie?   *1 mark*

Q 3. Where does the oesophagus enter the abdominal cavity?   *1 mark*

Q 4. What anatomical and physiological arrangements protect against gastro-oesophageal reflux?   *2 marks*

Because of his age, Mr Anderson was referred for further investigation. Upper GI endoscopy and barium swallow were carried out. Barium swallow revealed a sliding hiatus hernia.

Q 5. What is a hiatus hernia? *1 mark*

Q 6. Describe the difference between a sliding hiatus hernia and a rolling hiatus hernia. *2 marks*

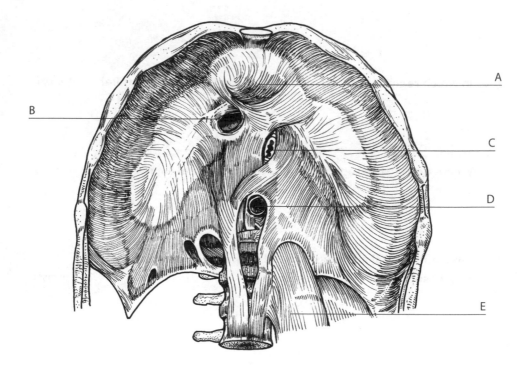

Figure 3.7: The diaphragm.

Q 7. On the opposite drawing of the diaphragm (Figure 3.7), identify A–E. *5 marks*

A –

B –

C –

D –

E –

Q 8. Label A–E on the following diagram (Figure 3.8). *2½ marks*

Choose from the following (½ mark for each):

- Chief cells.
- Gastric gland.
- Mucous neck cells.
- Gastric pit.
- Parietal cells.

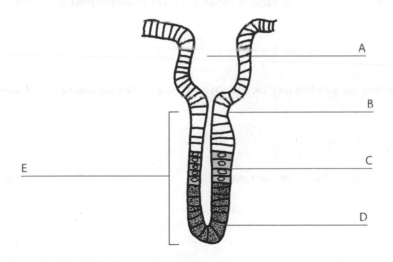

Figure 3.8: Epithelial cells of the stomach

A –

B –

C –

D –

E –

Q 9. What type of cell is found on the mucosal surface of the stomach lumen?   *½ mark*

Q 10. Which of the cell types in the gastric mucosa secretes hydrochloric acid?   *1 mark*

Q 11. Which cell type in the gastric mucosa secretes pepsinogen?   *1 mark*

Q 12. Which cell type in the gastric mucosa secretes intrinsic factor?   *1 mark*

Q 13. Why is intrinsic factor important?   *1 mark*

Q 14(a). Describe the mechanism of acid secretion in the stomach. *2 marks*

Q 14(b). Name four mediators that augment acid secretion. *2 marks*

During the upper GI endoscopy, the oesophagogastric junction was visualised. It revealed gastro-oesophageal reflux disease (GORD) with no complications.

Q 15. What type of epithelium lines the oesophagus? *1 mark*

The endoscopy report also mentioned that there was no evidence of 'the metaplastic changes of Barrett's oesophagus'.

Q 16. What is 'metaplasia'? *1 mark*

Q 17. What is the clinical significance of Barrett's oesophagus? *1 mark*

It is decided that Mr Anderson should be managed non-surgically with regular follow-up. You advise him on lifestyle changes, including cessation of smoking, limitation of large meals and eating near bedtime, and raising the head of the bed at night. You also prescribe some drugs.

Q **18. Name three drugs that can be used to manage a patient with gastro-oesophageal reflux disease and describe their mechanisms of action.**

3 marks

Drug	Mechanism of action

📖 **BIBLIOGRAPHY**

Kumar P, Clark M. 2005. *Clinical Medicine*, 6th edn. Edinburgh: Elsevier Saunders.

Standring S. 2005. *Gray's Anatomy*, 39th edn. Edinburgh: Elsevier Churchill Livingstone.

Widmaier EP, Raff H, Strang KT. 2006. *Vander's Human Physiology: the Mechanisms of Body Function*, 10th edn. Boston: McGraw Hill.

GASTROENTEROLOGY

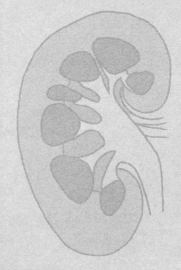

NEPHROLOGY CASE: QUESTIONS

NEPHROLOGY
1. CHRONIC RENAL FAILURE

Mr Shilliday is a pleasant 72-year-old man who comes to see you at the GP surgery because of a 2-month history of non-specific symptoms that include increasing tiredness, loss of appetite and generally feeling not quite himself. His skin is very itchy. You last saw him 1 year ago when he was very well.

The practice nurse takes a blood sample to check his liver function tests, his urea and electrolytes and his full blood count. You ask him to return in 48 hours.

These investigations reveal the following results:

FBC:
- **Haemoglobin – 7 (13–18 g/dl)**
- **MCV – 83 (76–96 fl)**
- **WCC – 8 [(4–11)×10^9/l]**
- **Platelets – 250 [(150–400)× 10^9/l]**

U&Es:

- **Na – 129 (135–145 mmol/l)**
- **K – 5.1 (3.5–5 mmol/l)**
- **Urea – 60 (2.5–6.7 mmol/l)**
- **Creatinine – 999 (70–150 µmol/l)**
- **Glucose – 5 (3.5–5.5 mmol/l)**
- **Ca – 1.6 (2.05–2.6 mmol/l)**
- **PO$_4{}^{2-}$ – 3.5 (0.8–1.4 mmol/l)**

LFTs

- **Albumin – 15 (35–50 g/l)**
- **Aspartate aminotransferase (AST) – 30 (3–35 iu/l)**
- **Alanine aminotransferase (ALT) – 20 (3–35 iu/l)**
- **Alkaline phosphatase – 300 (30–35 iu/l)**

NEPHROLOGY

From these results you suspect that he has chronic renal failure (CRF).

Q 1. List six results, which are strongly in keeping with this diagnosis, apart from raised serum creatinine and hypocalcaemia. *3 marks*

You ask the medical student who has been placed with you what she thinks of the results. Using her knowledge of renal physiology you ask her to explain the following.

Q 2. Why is serum creatinine a good marker of glomerular filtration rate? *2 marks*

It is apparent from the results of his FBC that Mr Shilliday has a normocytic, normochromic anaemia.

Q 3. Explain how this has come about. *2 marks*

Q 4. Explain the origin of the hypocalcaemia. *2 marks*

Since she has answered so well you try some basic anatomy questions!

Q 5. Name the structures indicated in the diagram below (Figure 4.1). *3 marks*

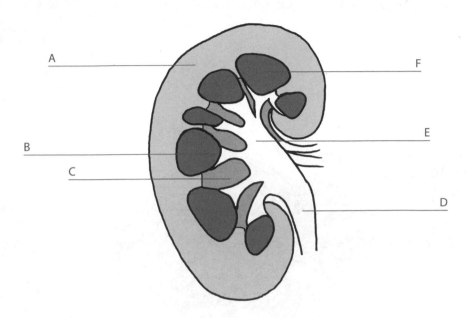

Figure 4.1: The kidney.

½ **mark for each of following:**

A –

B –

C –

D –

E –

F –

Q 6. Name structures A–D on the diagram (Figure 4.2) shown below of a
normal glomerulus.

4 marks

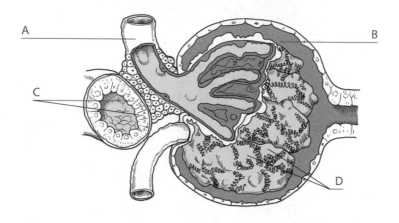

A

B

C

D

Figure 4.2: The normal glomerulus.

Q 7. List three other tests, apart from blood tests, which you could
now organise yourself in order to determine the cause of Mr Shilliday's
CRF.

3 marks

Test	Mark	Finding suggestive of CRF	Mark
	½		½
	½		½
	½		½

NEPHROLOGY

In view of his advanced CRF, however, you decide to refer Mr Shilliday as soon as possible to the local renal unit to be looked after by the renal physicians. He tells you that he has been suffering from some 'aches and pains' in the last couple of months. You suspect this is most likely due to renal osteodystrophy.

Q 8. What is meant by renal osteodystrophy?   *1 mark*

Q 9. Explain with the aid of a diagram the metabolism of vitamin D.   *4 marks*

At the local renal unit, biochemical investigation is carried out, which shows that Mr Shilliday has multiple myeloma, a malignant condition of red bone marrow. This is likely to be the cause his renal failure.

Q 10. Name the areas of the body where red bone marrow is found in the adult.   *2 marks*

Q **11. Name the specific abnormality that can be found in the urine in myeloma.** *1 mark*

Q **12. In the table below list three other tests that can be done to confirm the diagnosis of multiple myeloma and list the abnormality found in each.** *3 marks*

Test	Mark	Result indicative of myeloma	Mark
	½		½
	½		½
	½		½

Mr Shilliday died 6 months later at home surrounded by his family.

📖 BIBLIOGRAPHY

Scottish Renal Registry. Available online at http://www.srr.scot.nhs.uk/ and, more specifically, at http://www.srr.scot.nhs.uk/Report2004/SRR_Report_2002_2004.pdf

Horton-Szar D, Harris K. (eds) 2007. *Renal and Urinary Systems. Crash Course*, 3rd edn. London: Mosby.

[a]H. Bence Jones (1814–1873), English physician and skilled chemist who pioneered a scientific approach to clinical problems. First to describe the abnormal protein found in the urine of patients with multiple myeloma. It is characterised by precipitation at 56°C and re-solution at 100°C.

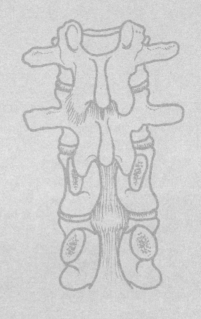

MUSCULOSKELETAL CASES:
QUESTIONS

MUSCULOSKELETAL
1. MUSCULAR DYSTROPHY

In the week after taking up a new appointment in orthopaedics, you are assisting at the outpatient clinic. One of the patients who attends is 28-year-old Mr Naismith. Before he arrives, you review the case notes. He has Becker's muscular dystrophy. You recall that this is a genetic disorder similar to Duchenne muscular dystrophy with the same form of inheritance. In Becker's muscular dystrophy reduced amounts of dystrophin are produced whereas in Duchenne muscular dystrophy very little is produced.

Q 1. What is the mode of inheritance of Becker's muscular dystrophy?   *1 mark*

Q 2. What is the function of dystrophin?   *1 mark*

Q 3. What is the name given to the basic functional unit of striated muscle?   *1 mark*

Q **4. On the following diagram (Figure 5.1) please label the following:** *2 marks*

A band

I band

Sarcomere

Z line

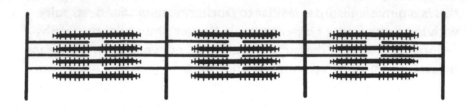

Figure 5.1: Striated muscle.

(2 marks – ½ mark for each.)

Q **5. What composes the thick and thin filaments?** *1 mark*

Thick filament		Thin filament	

Contraction of striated muscle is brought about by a mechanism sometimes known as the 'cross-bridge cycle'.

Q **6. What forms the 'cross-bridge'?** *1 mark*

Q 7. Describe the 'cross-bridge cycle'.   *4 marks*

Mr Naismith comes in using crutches. He has been unable to walk unaided for the last 18 months, the dystrophy in his lower limbs having become progressively worse since his late teens. The current problem is that he is on a follow-up visit after a fall four weeks ago. He fell on a step and landed awkwardly striking his right shoulder against a railing. The notes indicated that the shoulder had been quite badly bruised over the acromion but radiology had excluded a fracture or dislocation.

Q 8. Of which bone is the acromion a part? What is the relationship of the acromion to the shoulder joint?   *1 mark*

Q 9. Which parts of which bones form the shoulder joint?   *2 marks*

Q 10. In which joint does the acromion participate?   *1 mark*

The concern that necessitated follow-up at the clinic was that Mr Naismith had a degree of muscular weakness in his right upper limb. At the time of the accident, it was unclear whether this had been caused by the accident or was an indication that his muscular dystrophy was starting to affect his upper limb.

The following report of the upper limb examination has been recorded by the consultant in the case notes.

- **Right upper limb: General poverty of shoulder movement. Weakness of flexion of the elbow and of supination. Wrist and finger movements normal. No sensory loss detected. Poor biceps reflex but triceps reflex normal.**
- **Left upper limb: No abnormalities detected.**

Q **11. Which muscles flex the elbow?**   *1 mark*

Q **12. Which muscle is the principal supinator?**   *1 mark*

You think about the brachial plexus and the peripheral nerves of the upper limb.

Q **13. On the following outline of the brachial plexus (Figure 5.2), label the following.**   *6 marks*

Ventral ramus of C7

Superior trunk of brachial plexus

Lateral cord of brachial plexus

Median nerve

Radial nerve

Ulnar nerve

MUSCULOSKELETAL

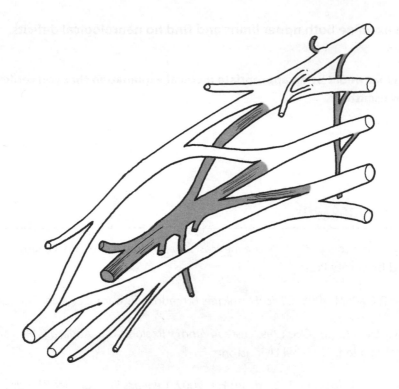

Figure 5.2: Brachial plexus.

Q 14. **Do you think the deficits recorded by the consultant suggest neurological damage or progression of the muscular dystrophy? Give reasons for your answer.** *6 marks*

You examine both upper limbs and find no neurological deficits.

Q 15. What would be an appropriate medical explanation that you could tell Mr Naismith. *1 mark*

📖 BIBLIOGRAPHY

Emery A, Muntoni F. 2003. *Duchenne Muscular Dystrophy*, 3rd edn. Oxford: Oxford University Press.

Kumar P, Clark M. 2005. *Clinical Medicine*, 6th edn. Edinburgh: Elsevier Saunders.

Last R J, Sinnatamby C S. 1999. *Last's Anatomy: Regional and Applied (MRCS Study Guides)*. London: Churchill Livingstone.

Nussbaum R L, McInnes R R, Willard H F. 2007. *Genetics in Medicine*, 7th edn. Philadelphia: Saunders.

Standring S. 2005. *Gray's Anatomy*, 39th edn. Edinburgh: Elsevier Churchill Livingstone.

Widmaier E P, Roff H, Strang K T. 2006. *Vander's Human Physiology. The Mechanism of Body Function*, 10th edn. Boston: McGraw Hill.

MUSCULOSKELETAL

MUSCULOSKELETAL
2. WRIST FRACTURE

Andrew Beattie, a 15-year-old boy, attends the Accident and Emergency Department after a fall at a school rugby match. He had fallen on his outstretched right hand. Movement at the wrist is limited and there is marked tenderness in the anatomical snuffbox. Radiology of the wrist is carried out and the following view obtained (Figure 5.3). The x-ray shows a fracture of the scaphoid bone.

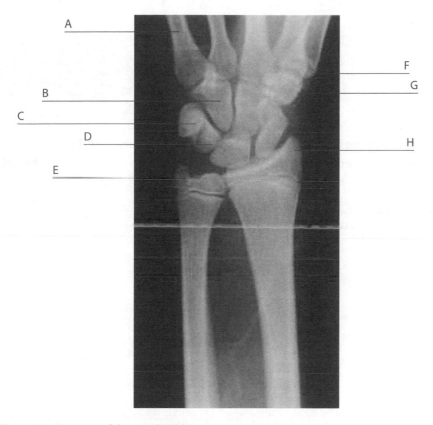

Figure 5.3: Fracture of the scaphoid bone

Q 1. Identify the structures labelled A–H in Figure 5.3. *4 marks*

½ mark for each:

A –

B –

C –

D –

E –

F –

G –

H –

Q 2. What structures form the medial and lateral boundaries of the anatomical snuffbox? *1 mark*

Medial boundary	
Lateral boundary	

Q 3. Andrew's wrist movement was limited. What movements normally occur at the wrist and which are the most restricted?   *4 marks*

Immobilisation in a plaster splint is required. The plaster is applied as far as the interphalangeal joint of the thumb and the metacarpophalangeal joints of the fingers. This supports the carpus while allowing movement of the thumb and fingers.

Q 4. To which varieties of synovial joints do these joints belong and what movements occur at them?   *2 marks*

Joint	Variety of synovial joint	Movement
Interphalangeal joint of thumb		
Metacarpophalangeal joint of finger		

Q 5. Only one muscle of the forearm attaches to a carpal bone. Which muscle is this and to which bone does it directly attach?   *2 marks*

Q **6. Explain how a fracture heals.** *6 marks*

Q **7. In the radiograph above (Figure 5.3), what are the radiolucent lines across the distal ends of the radius and the ulna and at the proximal end of the first metacarpal?** *1 mark*

Q **8. Why are such regions not visible in the second to fifth metacarpals in the above radiograph?** *1 mark*

Q **9. Chondrocytes are found in these radiolucent regions. What changes do these cells undergo at these sites?** *4 marks*

MUSCULOSKELETAL

Q 10. Define the terms 'diaphysis' and 'metaphysis'.   *2 marks*

Q 11. The ossification centres of the hand are useful in forensic work for establishing the age of juvenile subjects. What stage of formation have the carpal bones reached at the time of birth?   *1 mark*

Following fracture at the waist of the scaphoid bone, part of the scaphoid bone may undergo avascular necrosis.

Q 12. Which part of the scaphoid bone is usually affected by avascular necrosis and why?   *2 marks*

📖 BIBLIOGRAPHY

Crawford Adams J. Hamblen D L. 1999. *Outline of Fractures*, 11th edn. Edinburgh: Churchill Livingstone.

Scheuer L, Black S. 2000. *Developmental Juvenile Osteology*. London: Elsevier Academic Press.

Scothorne R J. 1976. Early development. In Passmore R, Robson J S (eds). *A Companion to Medical Studies*, 2nd edn., Vol. 1, chapter 19. Oxford: Blackwell Scientific Publications.

Solomon L, Warwick D, Nayagam S. 2001. *Apley's System of Orthopaedics and Fractures*, 8th edn. London: Arnold.

MUSCULOSKELETAL

MUSCULOSKELETAL
3. SPINE

Mr Martin, a 30-year-old teacher, has presented with low back pain of sudden onset. Over the school holidays he has been building a garden wall. The back pain came on when he attempted to lift a bag of cement. There was also a sensation of 'something giving'. The pain is in his lower back and is radiating to the perineum and down the backs of both thighs towards his calves. Mr Martin complains that the pain in his legs feels worse than that in his back. There is also a sensation of tingling down the back of the thigh and he has noticed that he has become numb at the lower part of his buttocks and around the region of his genitalia and anus. He has become incontinent of faeces and has not passed urine in the two hours since the injury.

Q 1. What is the most likely diagnosis for Mr Martin?   *2 mark*

On examination, sensory loss is detected on the back of both thighs and across the perineum. Motor function of both his lower limbs is difficult to assess because of the pain, but Mr Martin seems to be having particular difficulty moving his ankles. Ankle jerk reflexes are diminished, although knee jerk reflexes seem normal. An attempt to lift each leg passively from the bed with Mr Martin supine, the straight leg raise test, is also painful. It is also noted that Mr Martin has a palpable urinary bladder but is unable to pass urine (urinary retention) for which a catheter is passed.

Q 2. Which spinal nerves are involved in the knee-jerk and ankle-jerk reflexes?

1 mark

Q 3. Why did the straight leg raise test elicit pain? *1 mark*

Q 4. On the basis of motor signs, which nerve roots are most likely to have been affected by the prolapsed disc? Give reasons for your answer. *3 marks*

Q 5. Involvement of which spinal nerves is suggested by the sensory loss? Give reasons for your answer. *2 marks*

Q 6. Are the root values suggested by the motor and sensory signs consistent with the positive straight leg raise test? *1 mark*

Q 7. Which component of the intervertebral disc is it that prolapses? *1 mark*

Q 8. Identify features A–F on the following diagram (Figure 5.4).   *3 marks*

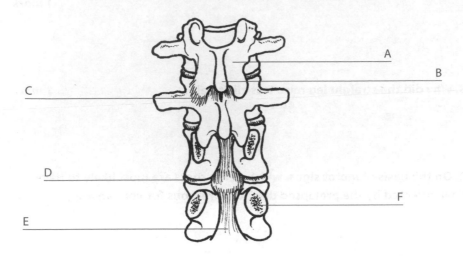

Figure 5.4: Anatomy of the spine.

½ mark for each:

A –

B –

C –

D –

E –

F –

In Mr Martin the disc has prolapsed centrally. It is more common (and less serious) for the disc to prolapse posterolaterally rather than passing directly posteriorly in the midline as in Mr Martin.

Q 9. Why does a disc tend to prolapse posterolaterally?   *2 marks*

Mr Martin is sent for an urgent MRI scan. The following is one of the images obtained (Figure 5.5).

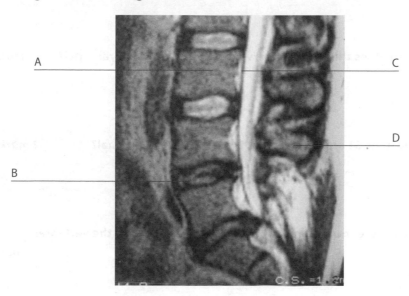

A

B

C

D

Figure 5.5: Mr Martin's MRI scan.

Q 10. On the image, identify A–D.   *4 marks*

1 mark for each:

A –

B –

C –

D –

Q 11. Which disc has prolapsed? *1 mark*

Q 12. Which component of the nervous system is found in the vertebral canal at this level? *1 mark*

Q 13. Where does the L4 spinal nerve exit from the vertebral canal? *1 mark*

Q 14. How does S1 spinal nerve exit from the vertebral canal? *2 marks*

Q 15. What is the lowest limit of the cerebrospinal fluid in the vertebral canal? *1 mark*

Q 16. Which nerves are responsible for maintenance of anal tone and what are their root values? *2 marks*

Q 17. Which nerves supply the detrusor muscle of the bladder? From which spinal nerves do they arise? *2 marks*

As a result of central prolapse pressing on the cauda equina, Mr Martin is diagnosed as having cauda equina syndrome and is referred for urgent neurosurgical decompression.

MUSCULOSKELETAL

📖 BIBLIOGRAPHY

Crawford Adams J. Hamblen D L. 2001. *Outline of Orthopaedics*, 13th edn. Edinburgh: Churchill Livingstone.

Ellis H. 2002. *Clinical Anatomy*, 10th edn. Oxford: Blackwell Publishing.

Solomon L, Warwick D, Nayagam S. 2001. *Apley's System of Orthopaedics and Fractures*, 8th edn. London: Arnold.

Standring S. 2005. *Gray's Anatomy*, 39th edn. Edinburgh: Elsevier Churchill Livingstone.

MUSCULOSKELETAL

MUSCULOSKELETAL
4. HERNIA

You are a surgical house officer and you are clerking in Mr Henderson who is being admitted for an elective open hernia repair.

While you are taking a history from Mr Henderson, he asks you what a hernia is.

Q **1. What is a hernia?** *1 mark*

Mr Henderson tells you that he was quite alarmed when he found a lump in his groin and was rather relieved when his GP told him it was a hernia and not something more serious.

Q **2. What is the differential diagnosis of a groin lump?** *3 marks*

Q **3. On your examination, how would you distinguish an inguinal hernia from a femoral hernia?** *2 marks*

You make a note that Mr Henderson has a right inguinal hernia. You also document that the hernia is 'reducible'.

Q 4. What does this term mean? *1 mark*

Q 5. List three complications of an irreducible hernia. Explain how they occur. *6 marks*

Complication	Marks	Explanation	Marks
	1		1
	1		1
	1		1

You wonder if it is a **direct** or an **indirect** inguinal hernia.

Q 6. How would you distinguish between these on clinical examination? *3 marks*

You are keen to pursue a career in surgery and manage to get time from your ward duties to observe Mr Henderson's operation in theatre. Your consultant, tells you that the femoral artery can be used as a landmark to determine the position of the deep inguinal ring.

Q 7. Where can the femoral artery be palpated? Give your answer in relation to bony landmarks. *1 mark*

Q 8. If inserting a needle into the femoral artery to collect arterial blood, it is important to appreciate the relationship of the femoral artery to the femoral nerve and femoral vein. What is this relationship? *1 mark*

Q 9. What is the position of the deep inguinal ring? Give your answer in relation to bony landmarks. *1 mark*

Q 10. What is the position of the deep ring in relation to the femoral artery? *1 mark*

Q 11. In this patient what structure passes through the deep inguinal ring that allows it to be easily identified by the surgeon? *1 mark*

The consultant continues to quiz your anatomical knowledge by asking you about the important structures in the inguinal canal.

Q 12. Name two structures in this patient's inguinal canal that a surgeon would take particular care to avoid damaging. *1 mark*

Q **13. Name four structures that lie within the spermatic cord.** *2 marks*

Q **14. Please identify structures A–H on this diagram (Figure 5.6) of the inguinal canal.** *4 marks*

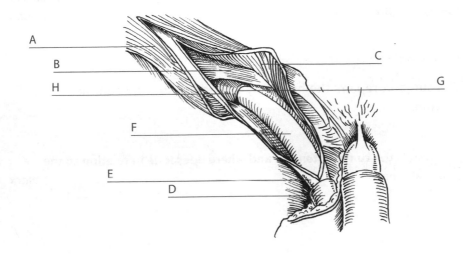

Figure 5.6: The Inguinal canal.

½ mark for each of the following:

A –

B –

C –

D –

E –

F –

G –

H –

Q 15. The hernial sac is found to lie medial to the inferior epigastric vessels. Is the hernia direct or indirect?   *1 mark*

The surgeon repairs the hernia by strengthening the conjoint tendon.

Q 16. What is the conjoint tendon and where does it lie in relation to the inguinal canal?   *1 mark*

📖 BIBLIOGRAPHY

Ellis H. 2002. *Clinical Anatomy*, 10th edn. Oxford: Blackwell Publishing.

Last R J, Sinnatamby C S. 1999. *Last's Anatomy: Regional and Applied*, 10th edn. Edinburgh: Churchill Livingstone.

Monkhouse S. 2001. *Clinical Anatomy*. Edinburgh: Churchill Livingstone.

MUSCULOSKELETAL
5. HIP FRACTURE

You are the Foundation Year 2 receiving doctor on the orthopaedic ward in a busy general hospital when Mrs Smith, a 76-year-old woman, is referred to you from the Accident and Emergency Department. Earlier in the day she had tripped on an uneven pavement and fallen on to her left side. She is now complaining of pain in her groin and thigh. The pain radiates to the knee. Mrs Smith is unable to weight-bear.

Q **1. From the history, what is the most likely diagnosis for Mrs Smith and explain your reasoning.** *2 marks*

An X-ray was taken (Figure 5.7) and the diagnosis confirmed.

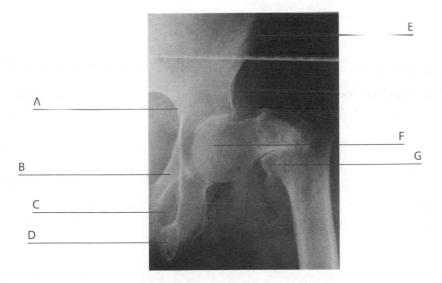

Figure 5.7: Mrs Smith's X-ray.

Q **2. Identify features A–G.**   *7 marks*

A –

B –

C –

D –

E –

F –

G –

The hip joint is innervated by branches of the femoral nerve, obturator nerve, accessory obturator nerve when present, and of the nerve to quadratus femoris. This helps explain the distribution of the pain.

Q **3. Why, as in Mrs Smith, does pain from the hip sometimes radiate to the knee?**   *1 mark*

Q **4. What is Hilton's Law[a]?**   *2 marks*

After a diagnosis has been established you start to consider whether there may be associated complications.

Q 5. List two acute complications that may follow fractured neck of femur. *2 marks*

Q 6. What is the main source of arterial blood supply of the head of the femur? *1 mark*

Q 7. What are the retinacular fibres of the hip joint capsule? *1 mark*

Q 8. What is their relationship to the blood supply of the head of the femur? *1 mark*

On further examination of Mrs Smith you find her left leg to be shortened and laterally (externally) rotated. This is due to muscle contraction.

Q 9. Name a muscle that laterally rotates the hip. *1 mark*

Mrs Smith had her hip surgically repaired by a hemiarthroplasty and began a programme of early mobilisation while recovering in hospital.

Q 10. What is a hemiarthroplasty?   *1 mark*

For one of the exercises, the physiotherapist told Mrs Smith to lie on her back, slide her foot up towards her buttock, bending her hip and knee (Figure 5.8).

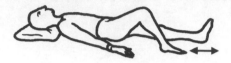

Figure 5.8: Physiotherapy exercises after hemiarthroplasty.

Q 11. Which muscle is the principal flexor of the hip?   *1 mark*

Q 12. Which three individual muscles are the principal flexors
of the knee?   *1½ marks*

Before Mrs Smith is discharged from hospital, she undergoes a dual-energy X-ray absorptiometry (DEXA) scan. It confirms that she is suffering from osteoporosis.

Q 13. Which cells of bone lay down new bone?   *½ mark*

Q 14. The table below indicates a number of features of osteocytes, osteoblasts and osteoclasts. In the right-hand column indicate of which cell type each of the features is characteristic.   *4 marks*

½ mark for each

Feature	Bone cell
Abundant lysosomes	
Abundant rough endoplasmic reticulum	
Basophilic cytoplasm	
Cellular processes in canaliculi	
Howship's lacuna	
Lie between bony lamellae	
Multiple nuclei	
Ruffled border	

Review of Mrs Smith's most recent post-operative blood results showed a profile compatible with a diagnosis of osteoporosis.

Q 15. Which of the following sets of results are Mrs Smith's? Explain your answer.   *2 marks*

	A	B	C	Normal range
Ca	2.3 mmol/l	2.5 mmol/l	1.9 mmol/l	2.20–2.67 mmol/l
PO_4	1.1 mmol/l	1.2 mmol/l	0.7 mmol/l	0.8–1.5 mmol/l
Alk. Phos.	1070 IU/ml	80 IU/l	205 IU/l	39–117 IU/l

Mrs Smith is prescribed calcium supplements and a bisphosphonate for her osteoporosis.

Q **16. How do bisphosphonates work?**   *2 marks*

📖 REFERENCES

Crawford Adams J. Hamblen D L. 1999. *Outline of Fractures*, 11th edn. Edinburgh: Churchill Livingstone.

Ellis H. 2002. *Clinical Anatomy*, 10th edn. Oxford: Blackwell Publishing.

Kumar P, Clark M. 2005. *Clinical Medicine*, 6th edn. Edinburgh: Elsevier Saunders.

Last R J, Sinnatamby C S. 1999. *Last's Anatomy: Regional and Applied*, 10th edn. Edinburgh: Churchill Livingstone.

Provan D, Krentz A. 2002. *Oxford Handbook of Clinical and Laboratory Investigation*. Oxford: Oxford University Press.

[a]John Hilton (1805–1934), surgeon at Guy's Hospital London, described the innervation of joints. He was President of the Royal College of Surgeons of England in 1867 and surgeon extraordinary to Queen Victoria.

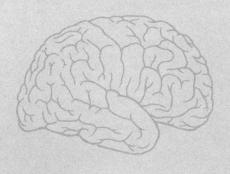

NEUROLOGY CASES:
QUESTIONS

NEUROLOGY
1. MOTOR NEURON DISEASE

You are on duty at a local hospice. 34-year-old Mr Wilson is admitted for one week of respite care. It is your duty to clerk him in. Mr Wilson was diagnosed with motor neuron disease 18 months ago.

Q 1. What is motor neuron disease? *½ mark*

Q 2. Which components of the central nervous system (CNS) are affected in motor neuron disease? *1½ marks*

Q 3. In which pathways from the motor cortex do most motor impulses descend? *1 mark*

Q 4. What is a motor unit? *1 mark*

Since motor neuron disease affects motor neurons, the clinical manifestations are primarily within skeletal muscles rather than in smooth or cardiac muscle.

Q 5. Complete the following table comparing the three muscle types. *6 marks*

	Skeletal	Cardiac	Smooth
Striated or non-striated?			
Peripheral or central nucleus/nuclei?			
Single or multiple nuclei?			
Small, large or very large fibre diameter?			

After taking a full and detailed history, you examine Mr Wilson. During the examination of the nervous system, you find that in Mr Wilson's upper limbs there are muscle wasting, fasciculation and reduced power in all muscle groups.

Q 6. What do the fasciculations indicate?   *1 mark*

You continue with the neurological examination and find there is also reduced power in the lower limbs.

Q 7. Identify the following features on the diagram (Figure 6.1) of the calf muscles of the right lower limb.   *3 marks*

A –

B –

C –

D –

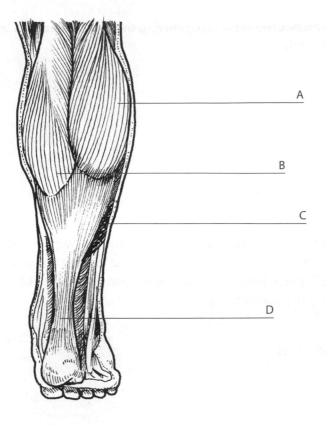

A

B

C

D

Figure 6.1: Anatomy of the calf muscles of the right lower limb.

After examining Mr Wilson you present your findings to the on-call consultant. You note that there was no involvement of the extraocular muscles. The consultant explains to you that in motor neuron disease the extraocular muscles are often not involved and, if they are, it is a very late feature of the disease. She also tells you that in patients with advanced motor neuron disease, movement of the eyeball is often the only means of communication. Special boards are used which allow the patient to spell out words by looking at letters on the board in order to communicate.

NEUROLOGY

Q **8. List the six muscles responsible for moving the eyeball and give the nerve supply of each.** *3 marks*

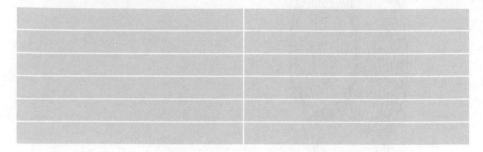

Mr Wilson's wife explains that a few months ago Mr Wilson lost the ability to chew and swallow safely. He had lost almost a stone in weight before a percutaneous endoscopic gastrostomy (PEG) tube was inserted by the surgical team.

Q **9. What is a PEG tube?** *1 mark*

Q **10. Identify the muscles that are shown in this illustration (Figure 6.2).** *2 marks*

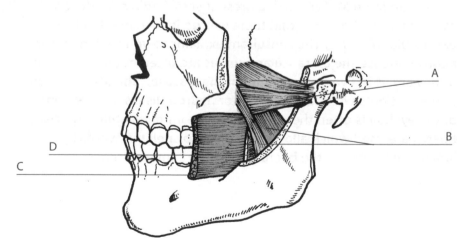

Figure 6.2: Some muscles of chewing and swallowing

½ mark for each of the following:

A –

B –

C –

D –

Q 11. What is the innervation of the 'muscles of mastication'?   *1 mark*

During examination of Mr Wilson's cranial nerves, you find abnormalities of the facial nerve. You find he can only raise his eyebrows minimally and not against resistance.

Q 12. Which muscle is responsible for raising the eyebrows?   *1 mark*

You notice that Mr Wilson is also unable to close his eyes tightly.

Q 13. Which muscle is responsible for this action?   *1 mark*

On further examination of the facial nerve you notice Mr Wilson has great difficulty when asked to 'blow out his cheeks'.

Q 14. Which muscle is being used in this part of the examination?   *1 mark*

NEUROLOGY

As well as supplying the muscles of facial expression, the facial nerve has sensory and autonomic functions.

Q 15. What are the sensory and autonomic functions of the facial nerve? *2 marks*

Nearing completion of your examination of the cranial nerves you find that Mr Wilson is unable to shrug his shoulders.

Q 16. Which cranial nerves are responsible for this action? *1 mark*

Q 17. The following diagram (Figure 6.3) shows the attachments of the cranial nerves to the brain. Identify structures A–F. *3 marks*

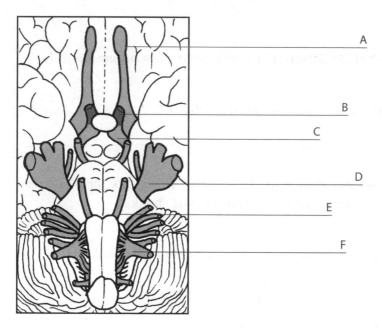

A

B

C

D

E

F

Figure 6.3: Attachments of the cranial nerves to the brain

NEUROLOGY

½ mark for each of the following:

A –

B –

C –

D –

E –

F –

📖 BIBLIOGRAPHY

Hiatt J L, Gartner L P. 2000. *Textbook of Head and Neck Anatomy*, 3rd edn. New York: Lippincott, Williams and Wilkins.

Johnson D R, Moore W J. 1997. *Anatomy for Dental Students*, 3rd edn. Oxford: Oxford University Press.

Kiernan J A. 2005. *Barr's The Human Nervous System: An Anatomical Viewpoint*, 8th edn. Philadelphia: Lippincott Williams and Wilkins.

Standring S. 2005. *Gray's Anatomy*, 39th edn. Edinburgh: Elsevier Churchill Livingstone.

Tortora G J, Grabowski S. 2002. *Principles of Anatomy and Physiology*, 10th edn. New York: John Wiley.

NEUROLOGY

NEUROLOGY
2. CEREBRAL ARTERY DISEASE

You are working in general practice when 61-year-old Mr Johnston comes to see you complaining of having 'funny turns' recently. He describes two episodes which occurred within the last three weeks. He explains that during the first episode the vision in his left eye became 'foggy' for about two minutes. During the next episode his vision 'went funny' again and he became weak down his right side. This also lasted a few minutes. Following both episodes Mr Johnston was well. Further questioning reveals that the weakness particularly affected his right hand and right lower limb. The visual disturbance in the second attack was not the same as in the first. The first time only Mr Johnston's left eye was affected and the sight was completely lost for the duration of the attack. The second time the attack affected both eyes and he seemed to lose the right side of his field of vision in both eyes.

Q 1. What is the most likely diagnosis of the first episode when Mr Johnston had visual impairment in his left eye?   *1 mark*

Q 2. What is the most likely diagnosis of the second episode?   *1 mark*

Q 3. Where are the sites of ischaemia likely to be in the first and second episodes? Explain your reasoning. *4 marks*

On examination, you find Mr Johnston to be well. He is a heavy man with central obesity and a ruddy complexion. His pulse is regular with a rate of 82 beats per minute and his blood pressure is 172/94 mmHg. You also notice that Mr Johnston has xanthelasma and corneal arcus, but there are no further cardiovascular findings to note. Neurological examination is normal.

Q 4. What is xanthelasma and what is its clinical significance? *1 mark*

Q 5. Is the corneal arcus (arcus senilis) significant? *1 mark*

NEUROLOGY

You start Mr Johnson on aspirin and after an ECG, repeat blood pressure measurements and carry out further assessment of his blood cholesterol/lipoprotein levels. You also prescribe a statin for his cholesterol and a thiazide diuretic for his blood pressure.

Q 6. Describe how these drugs work.   *3 marks*

1 mark per drug

Drug	Mechanism of action
Aspirin	
Statin	
Thiazide diuretic	

Mr Johnston also has carotid Doppler[a] ultrasound studies which show stenosis at the lower end of the left internal carotid.

Q 7. What arteries arise from the internal carotid artery in the cranial cavity?   *4 marks*

_____

_____

_____

_____

Q 8. On the following diagram (Figure 6.4) indicate the location of:

    the central sulcus
    the lateral fissure
    the primary motor cortex

Indicate the regions of the motor cortex that serve:
the upper limb
the lower limb
the head and neck

6 marks

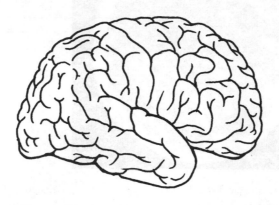

Figure 6.4: Surface anatomy of the brain.

Q 9. In neuroanatomy, what is meant by the term somatotopic localisation?

1 mark

Mr Johnston is referred to the vascular surgeons.

You recall seeing a patient when you worked in hospital where undetected embolic disease resulted in a stroke. The 70-year-old patient presented with a left hemiplegia. One of the CT scan views is shown overleaf (Figure 6.5).

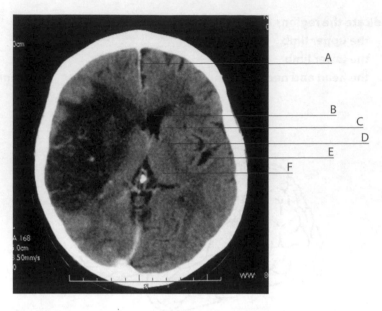

Figure 6.5: CT scan.

Q 10. On the CT scan identify A–F.   *6 marks*

A –

B –

C –

D –

E –

F –

Q 11. Why did this patient have a left hemiplegia?   *2 marks*

📖 BIBLIOGRAPHY

Axford J, O'Callaghan C. 2004. *Medicine*, 2nd edn. Oxford: Blackwell.

Fitzgerald M J T, Hruener G, Mtui E. 2007. *Clinical Neuroanatomy and Neuroscience*. Philadelphia: Elsevier Saunders.

Kiernan J A. 2005. *Barr's The Human Nervous System: An Anatomical Viewpoint*, 8th edn. Philadelphia: Lippincott Williams and Wilkins.

Kumar P, Clark M. 2005. *Clinical Medicine*, 6th edn. Edinburgh: Elsevier Saunders.

[a]Christian Doppler (1803–1853), Austrian mathematician and physicist, who described the Doppler effect, the apparent change in frequency and wavelength of a wave as perceived by an observer moving relative to the source of the wave.

NEUROLOGY

NEUROLOGY
3. MULTIPLE SCLEROSIS

You are a GP waiting on your final patient on a busy Friday afternoon. You check the computer screen and see that it is a 28-year-old woman, Miss Fraser. You are well acquainted with Miss Fraser as she has been attending your practice frequently over the past few months following a diagnosis of multiple sclerosis.

Multiple sclerosis is a disease characterised by demyelination of the neurones within the central nervous system (CNS).

Q 1. **Which cells are responsible for myelin production in the CNS and in the peripheral nervous system (PNS)?** *1 mark*

Q 2. **Label this diagram (Figure 6.6) of a neuron.** *3 marks*

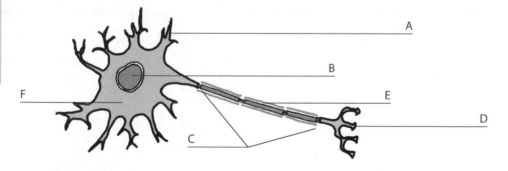

Figure 6.6: A neuron.

½ mark for each of the following:

A –

B –

C –

D –

E –

F –

Q 3. Give three ways in which a (lower) motor neuron differs from a sensory neuron. *3 marks*

When you last saw Miss Fraser she had been complaining of reduced vision and pain in her right eye. During your examination at the time, you noted that her right pupil was constricting further when you shone a light into her left eye than when you shone light into the right eye directly.

Q 4. What is the name of this phenomenon? *1 mark*

Q 5. Describe the steps of the normal pupillary light reflex when a light is shone into the eye. *3 marks*

This time, Miss Fraser enters the room and sits down. She tells you that her eye pain has now gone.

'I don't understand doctor, I thought multiple sclerosis was a progressive illness, how can my eyes get better?' You explain to Miss Fraser that this is due to the type of MS she has.

Q 6. Explain three of the different forms of multiple sclerosis.   *3 marks*

Unfortunately, Miss Fraser has not been doing so well. She tells you that she has noticed weakness of her legs and feels like she always needs to use the bathroom. She asks you if this could be due to her MS. You explain that MS commonly involves the spinal cord and the symptoms she is describing are indicative of this.

Q 7. What is the name given to spinal cord involvement in multiple sclerosis?   *1 mark*

Q 8. What clinical signs indicate that multiple sclerosis is affecting the spinal cord?   *3 marks*

Q **9. Label the following features on this diagram (Figure 6.7) of a sagittal section through the brainstem and cerebellum.**

3 marks (½ mark for each item)

Cerebral aqueduct

Cerebellar tonsil

Fourth ventricle

Medulla oblongata

Pons

White matter of the cerebellum

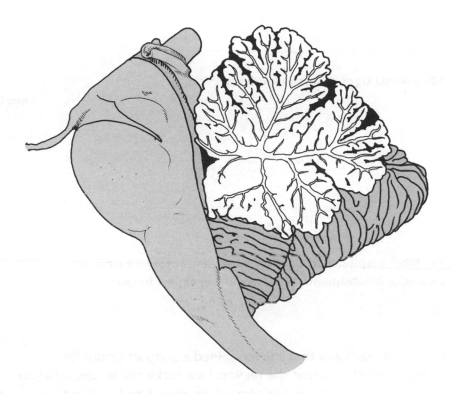

Figure 6.7: Sagittal section through brainstem and cerebellum.

Q 10. Name the ridges on the surface of the cerebellum. *1 mark*

Q 11. Name the principal nucleus that lies within the cerebellar hemisphere. *1 mark*

Q 12. Name the bundles that connect the cerebellum to the midbrain, the pons and the medulla respectively. *1 mark*

Q 13. Give six signs of cerebellar dysfunction.

3 marks

Q 14. What hospital investigation would confirm your suspicions of cerebellar involvement? What would you expect to see? *1 mark*

Miss Fraser tells you that she has joined a support group for sufferers of MS and that she realises how lucky she is. She tells you that some of the people are wheelchair-bound and unable to move their legs.

You recall that MS affecting the spinal cord can cause an upper motor neuron lesion.

NEUROLOGY

Q 15. What are the clinical features of an upper motor neurone lesion?

2 marks

📖 BIBLIOGRAPHY

Compston A, Confavreux C, Lassmann H, McDonald I R, Miller D H, Noseworthy J, Smith K J, Wekerle H. 2006. *McAlpine's Multiple Sclerosis*, 4th edn. Philadelphia: Churchill Livingstone Elsevier.

Holmes O. 1993. *Human Neurophysiology: A Student Text*, 2nd edn. London: Chapman and Hall Medical.

Kiernan J A. 2005. *Barr's The Human Nervous System: An Anatomical Viewpoint*, 8th edn. Philadelphia: Lippincott Williams and Wilkins.

NEUROLOGY
4. SPINAL CORD COMPRESSION

Miss Hunter is a 38-year-old woman with a known history of breast cancer. She was diagnosed after finding a lump in her right breast 3 years ago. This was identified as a ductal carcinoma-in-situ and was removed with breast conservation, a wide local excision and lymph node dissection. The pathologist reported the cancer as:

- invasive carcinoma, Grade 2, with a maximal diameter of 24 mm
- surgical margins clear of disease
- oestrogen receptor-negative
- metastatic disease in 3 of 16 lymph nodes.

Miss Hunter then underwent radiotherapy and chemotherapy.

Q 1. Mammary glands are specialised accessory glands of the skin. Name four general types of gland associated with the skin. *2 marks*

Q 2. Label the following diagram (Figure 6.8) showing the basic structure of the breast. *3 marks*

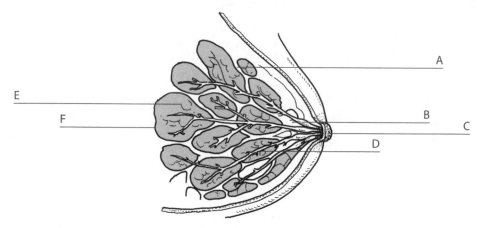

Figure 6.8: Basic anatomy of the breast.

½ mark for each correct label:

A –

B –

C –

D –

E –

F –

After birth, a hormone secreted from the anterior pituitary gland stimulates milk production.

Q 3. What is this hormone called? *1 mark*

Suckling causes the pituitary gland to release oxytocin, which causes the myoepithelial cells to contract.

Q 4. From which part of the pituitary does it come? *1 mark*

Q 5. Where is oxytocin produced? *1 mark*

Q 6. Where in the breast are myoepithelial cells found? *1 mark*

Q 7. What is the function of a myoepithelial cell within the breast? *1 mark*

Miss Hunter has a family history of breast cancer. Her grandmother was diagnosed with breast cancer aged 42. Miss Hunter's mother's elder sister (Miss Hunter's aunt) was diagnosed with breast cancer aged 38. Miss Hunter's elder sister was diagnosed with ovarian cancer last year, aged 42; her younger sister is healthy aged 36. Miss Hunter's mother has not had any cancer and is still healthy aged 66. There is no history of breast or ovarian cancer on Miss Hunter's father's side of the family.

Q 8. Please draw a family tree illustrating Miss Hunters relevant family history, indicating the age at diagnosis of those individuals affected. *3 marks*

Q 9. Which two genes are most strongly associated with *both* breast and ovarian cancer? *1 mark*

Three years later, Miss Hunter has now presented to you, her GP, with a 24-hour history of back pain. She has no history of recent injury. She has been feeling lethargic and has lost 3 kg over the last month. You notice as she walks into your surgery that she appears to have an ataxic gait. You are concerned that this could be the start of spinal cord compression and send Miss Hunter straight to hospital for urgent assessment.

NEUROLOGY

Q 10. What is the most likely cause of spinal cord compression in a patient with this history? *1 mark*

Q 11. Through which opening in the base of the skull is the spinal cord continuous with the brain stem? *1 mark*

Q 12. At what vertebral level does the spinal cord end? *1 mark*

Q 13. What is the name of the collection of nerve roots that continue down in the lumbar region of the spinal canal? *1 mark*

Q 14. Below is a diagram (Figure 6.9) of a thoracic vertebra. Identify A–F. *3 marks*

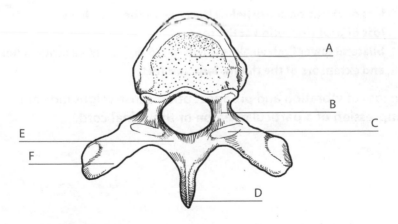

Figure 6.9: The thoracic vertebra.

½ mark for each correct label:

A –

B –

C –

D –

E –

F –

Q 15. At each spinal level, a pair of spinal nerves emerges from the intervertebral foramina. What connects each of these spinal nerves to the spinal cord?   *1 mark*

Miss Hunter arrives at the hospital where the receiving doctor agrees a diagnosis of spinal cord compression is possible. He conducts a neurological examination which now shows:

- loss of vibration sense below the level of the umbilicus
- loss of proprioception at the toes
- bilateral lower limb weakness with a 3/5 degree of severity in flexors and extensors of the thighs, legs and feet.

The loss of vibration and proprioception sense might indicate compression of a particular region of the spinal cord.

Q 16. On the diagram below (Figure 6.10), please shade the area of the tracts whose compression is most likely to cause loss of vibration and proprioception. *1 mark*

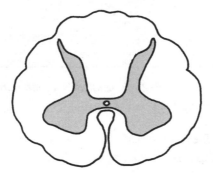

Figure 6.10: Transverse section of spinal cord.

Q 17. Loss of vibration sensation below the level of the umbilicus would indicate a spinal cord compression at what spinal level? *1 mark*

Q 18. Please fill in the table below. *6 marks*

Pathway	Ascending/descending?	What modalities/functions are mediated via the pathway?
Lateral corticospinal tract		
Dorsal column/medial lemniscus pathway		
Spinothalamic tract		
Spinocerebellar tract		

Spinal cord compression is an oncological emergency and a steroid therapy was started and imaging arranged to assess the appropriateness of surgery and radiotherapy in treatment.

📖 BIBLIOGRAPHY

Fitzgerald M J T, Hruener G, Mtui E. 2007. *Clinical Neuroanatomy and Neuroscience*. Philadelphia: Elsevier Saunders.

Kiernan J A. 2005. *Barr's The Human Nervous System: An Anatomical Viewpoint*, 8th edn. Philadelphia: Lippincott Williams and Wilkins.

Nussbaum R L, McInnes R R, Willard H F. 2007. *Genetics in Medicine*, 7th edn. Philadelphia: Saunders.

NEUROLOGY

NEUROLOGY
5. STROKE

Mr McKay is a 68-year-old man who is attending a routine check up at his local GP practice. He has no symptoms and urine dipstick test is negative. His blood pressure is 155/98 mmHg and he has a body mass index (BMI) of 30 kg/m².

Q 1. How do you routinely measure systolic and diastolic blood pressure using a stethoscope?   *2 marks*

Q 2. Prior to treatment, what would you do next with regard to this blood pressure result?   *1 mark*

Q 3. What is the equation for calculating mean arterial pressure from the measured pressures?   *1 mark*

Q 4. How is body mass index calculated?   *1 mark*

Q 5. Into what body mass index category would the following patients fall?   *1 mark*

Q 5(a). A man with BMI index = 15.0 kg/m².

Q 5(b). A woman with BMI = 35.0 kg/m².

The GP later decides to treat Mr McKay's raised blood pressure. Mr McKay is unhappy, however, as he feels fit and healthy and asks why he is being put on medication when he feels well.

Q 6. Suggest three advantages/reasons for Mr McKay being put on medication to control his hypertension. *2 marks*

Q 7. Give three classes of drug commonly used in the treatment of hypertension. For each class, briefly describe their mechanism of action. *6 marks*

1 mark for each class of drug and for its mechanism:

Type of drug	Mechanism of action

Mr McKay is concerned about the side-effects. He describes having a friend who is on treatment for hypertension and suffers from dizzy spells when standing up. This is postural hypotension.

Q 8. When a healthy person stands up what physiological mechanism maintains/restores blood pressure? *2 marks*

Q 9. Explain the physiological mechanism by which postural hypotension occurs. *1½ marks*

Q 10. In a healthy young adult, which is more noticeable on moving from a lying to a standing position – a fall in blood pressure or a rise in heart rate? *½ mark*

Several weeks later you are called by Mr McKay's wife who came home from shopping and found him collapsed on the floor. He is very confused and his speech sounds abnormal. He also has an obvious weakness on the right side of his body. You suspect he has had a stroke.

You note that Mr McKay has an irregular pulse. Upon further examination you find Mr McKay has trouble comprehending spoken and written language, producing coherent speech, and has paralysis on the right side in his upper limb and face but not in his lower limb.

NEUROLOGY

Q **11. What are the two specific areas in the brain concerned with speech and what language problems can result from damage to these areas?** *2 marks*

Q **12. Identify A–H on the diagram (Figure 6.11) of the circle of Willis[a] and the major arteries supplying the brain.** *4 marks*

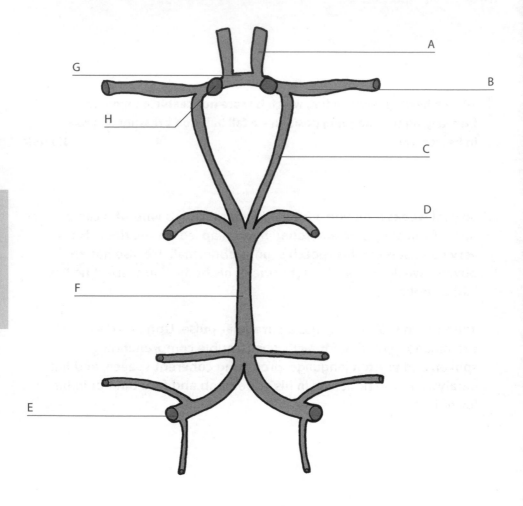

Figure 6.11: Circle of Willis.

NEUROLOGY

½ mark for each artery:

A –

B –

C –

D –

E –

F –

G –

H –

Q 13. Blockage of which artery is most likely to explain this man's symptoms?   *1 mark*

Mr McKay arrives in hospital. A CT scan of his brain shows an area of ischaemia in the regions of the left hemisphere adjacent to the lateral fissure, and an ECG shows atrial fibrillation (AF).

Q 14. On the following diagram (Figure 6.12) indicate the territories of the cerebral arteries.   *3 marks*

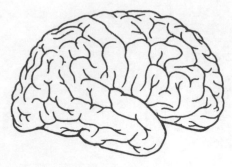

Figure 6.12: Territories of the cerebral arteries.

(1 mark for accurate representation of the territory supplied by each cerebral artery)

Q 15. Of the clinical information gathered on the patient to date, what is the most likely explanation of why he has had a stroke?   *2 marks*

📖 **BIBLIOGRAPHY**

Axford J, O'Callaghan C. 2004. *Medicine*, 2nd edn. Oxford: Blackwell.

Fitzgerald M J T, Hruener G, Mtui E. 2007. *Clinical Neuroanatomy and Neuroscience*. Philadelphia: Elsevier Saunders.

Kiernan J A. 2005. *Barr's The Human Nervous System: An Anatomical Viewpoint*, 8th edn. Philadelphia: Lippincott Williams and Wilkins.

Widmaier E P, Roff H, Strang K T. 2006. *Vander's Human Physiology. The Mechanism of Body Function*, 10th edn. Boston: McGraw Hill.

[a]Thomas Willis (1621–1675), English physician, who described the circulus arteriosus cerebri and was a founder of the Royal Society.

NEUROLOGY

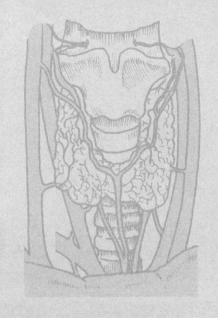

ENDOCRINOLOGY CASES: QUESTIONS

ENDOCRINOLOGY
1. ADDISON'S DISEASE

You are a junior doctor in Accident and Emergency when one Saturday morning 58-year-old Mr Gordon is rushed in. He was found by his wife, who has followed the ambulance to the hospital. She is very anxious and struggles to give a clear history. Mr Gordon has reduced consciousness and appears to be seriously unwell.

You begin an initial assessment and discover that Mr Gordon is cold and clammy with a blood pressure of 90/60 mmHg and a heart rate of 140 beats per minute, leading you to consider that he might be in shock.

As you begin a more thorough examination, you discover a silver bracelet (Figure 7.1) around his wrist with the following symbol.

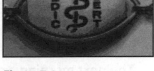

Figure 7.1

On noticing this you question Mrs Gordon (who has now calmed down) about her husband's medical history and medication, and discover that Mr Gordon was diagnosed with Addison's disease[a] 5 months ago and started on daily corticosteroid replacement therapy.

Q 1. What is Addison's disease?   *1 mark*

Addison's disease is relatively rare: with a prevalence of about 4 per 100 000 people in the UK.

Q 2. What is the main aetiology in affluent countries?   *1 mark*

ENDOCRINOLOGY

Mrs Gordon also tells you that a fortnight ago her husband was an in-patient and was diagnosed with severe community-acquired pneumonia, and treated with amoxicillin.

His respiratory symptoms have now subsided, but over the last few days he has been vomiting and has been 'off his food'. His temperature has been around 38°C, and he has been complaining of generalised abdominal pain, weakness and dizziness, especially when he tries to stand. Mrs Gordon has also noticed a change in mood, her husband having become somewhat apathetic. More worryingly, he has become acutely confused within the last 24 hours.

Q 3. What drug would you administer now and how?   *2 marks*

The next morning a short synacthen test was performed.

Mr Gordon's results:

Time (min)	Cortisol level in Mr Gordon's serum (nmol/l)	Normal serum levels throughout test (nmol/l)
0	90	> 170
30	90	> 580

Q 4. Explain Mr Gordon's low baseline serum cortisol level (time 0) and why his body does not respond to the synacthen test (+ 30 min).   *2 marks*

The adrenals (suprarenals) are endocrine glands located at the superior poles of the kidneys. The left is crescentic and the right tetrahedral in shape.

Q **5. Identify A–C in the diagram below (Figure 7.2).**   *1 mark*

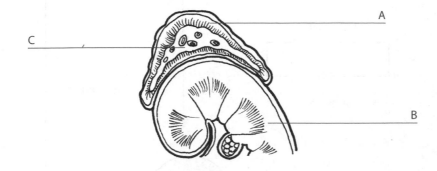

Figure 7.2: Adrenal gland.

A – _____

B – _____

C – _____

Q **6. Name the three zones of the adrenal cortex and the hormone produced from each of these areas.**   *3 marks*

Zone of adrenal cortex	Hormone

Q **7. The adrenal medulla is also a site of hormone secretion: name its products.**   *1 mark*

Q 8. Complete the diagram (Figure 7.3) below illustrating the homeostatic control of cortisol release. **3 marks**

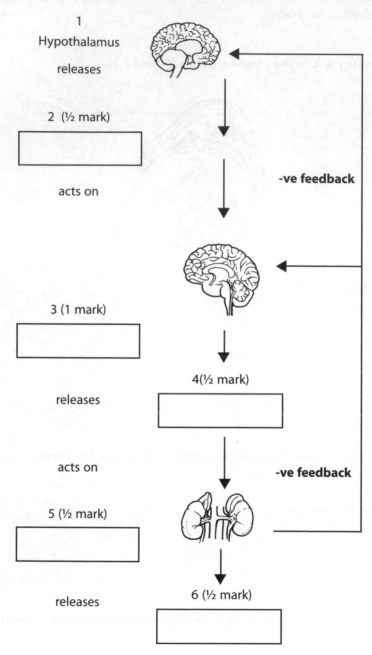

Figure 7.3: Homeostatic control of cortisol release.

The diagram below (Figure 7.4) shows the pituitary gland, composed of two lobes and connected to the hypothalamus by the pituitary stalk, which contains both nerve fibres and blood vessels.

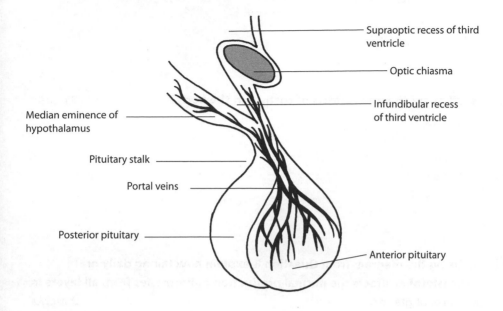

Figure 7.4: The pituitary gland.

Q 9. Which lobe of the pituitary is connected to the hypothalamus by blood vessels? *1 mark*

Q 10. Name these vessels. *1 mark*

Q 11. Which hormones travel to the pituitary gland via nerve fibres? *1 mark*

Q 12. Which hormones are produced by the anterior pituitary?   *3 marks*

Q 13. What are the main effects of cortisol in the body?   *3 marks*

Q 14. Using the diagram from Question 8 explain how taking daily oral corticosteroids affects the normal production of hormones from all layers in the adrenal glands.   *2 marks*

Mr Gordon's hospital case notes have now arrived. Prior to his initial diagnosis of Addison's disease, Mr Gordon had experienced loss of appetite, nausea, occasional vomiting and weight loss. He felt weak and somewhat depressed and complained of being suddenly dizzy on standing up. Moreover he had noticed patches of dull/grey discoloration appearing mainly on areas exposed to both light and pressure: his elbows, knuckles, palmar creases, and also on a recent scar on his left knee

Q 15. Explain the cause of these pigmentation patches. *1 mark*

Q 16. In which layer of the skin are the melanocytes found? *1 mark*

The next day the results of Mr Gordon's blood tests taken on admission become available.

	Mr Gordon's serum levels	Normal range
Na$^+$	80 mmol/l	135–145 mmol/l
K$^+$	6.7 mmol/l	3.5–5.0 mmol/l
Blood glucose (fasting)	2.5 mmol/l	3.5–5.5 mmol/l
Urea	18.0 mmol/l	2.5–6.7 mmol/l
Creatinine	178 µmol/l	70–150 µmol/l

Q 17. Explain these biochemical abnormalities. *2 marks*

Mr Gordon is also taking 75 µg fludrocortisone twice daily.

Q 18. What is this drug and why is it important in the treatment of Addison's disease? *1 mark*

After 48 h Mr Gordon has been stabilised and is moved to the medical ward for monitoring until he is fit to go home.

On discharge Mr and Mrs Gordon thank the hospital staff for their care. You warn Mr Gordon again about the seriousness of this situation, and how lucky he has been on this occasion. Careful attention must be given to avoid a similar episode happening again and he must always remember to wear his 'Medic Alert' bracelet.

📖 BIBLIOGRAPHY

Besser G M, Thorner M O. 2002. *Comprehensive Clinical Endocrinology*, 3rd edn. London: Mosby.

Greenspan F S, Stewler G J. 1997. *Basic and Clinical Endocrinology*, 5th edn. London: Prentice Hall.

[a]Thomas Addison (1793–1860). An Edinburgh graduate (1815), Addison became a physician and lecturer in Materia Medica at Guy's Hospital, London, where he was a skilful diagnostician. He committed suicide at the age of 67, having been forced to retire because of melancholia.

ENDOCRINOLOGY

ENDOCRINOLOGY
2. DIABETES MELLITUS

You are the receiving physician in the Accident and Emergency Department. Miss Winters is a 23-year-old engineering student who presents drowsy and confused. Her sister has brought her in and tells you that Miss Winters has been an insulin-dependent diabetic since childhood. For the past 2 days Miss Winters has had 'food poisoning'. Miss Winters's heart rate is 116 beats per minute and her blood pressure is 95/60 mmHg. There is reduced skin turgor and her tongue is dry.

Q 1. Which cells secrete insulin and to which group of cells in the pancreas do they belong?   *1 mark*

Q 2. Precisely how do the cells that secrete insulin react to increasing concentrations of circulating glucose?   *3 marks*

Q 3. What is the general structure of the human insulin molecule in the bloodstream?   *1 mark*

Q 4. What protein, secreted with insulin, can be used as a marker for insulin production?   *1 mark*

Q 5. Describe the transduction of the insulin signal in the effector cell.   *4 marks*

Q 6. Is Miss Winters likely to be a type I or type II diabetic?   *1 mark*

Q 7. Which form of diabetes is usually an HLA-associated autoimmune disease?   *1 mark*

Q 8. What would be an appropriate adjustment to an insulin regime during a period of intercurrent illness and why?   *1 mark*

Miss Winters is still drowsy and taking deep sighing breaths despite oxygen. A finger-prick sample of blood shows that her glucose level is 25 mmol/l and her urine is positive for ketones and glucose.

ENDOCRINOLOGY

Q 9. What is the name given to the hyperventilation that Miss Winters is demonstrating? *1 mark*

Q 10. Which three ketones are produced during diabetic ketoacidosis? *1 mark*

Q 11. Explain how insulin deficiency results in ketone production. *3 marks*

You take an arterial blood gas sample. The results are:

Parameter	Miss Winters' value	Normal range
pH	7.05	7.35–7.45
$[H^+]$ (nmol/l)	90	35–45
$[HCO_3^-]$ (mmol/l)	8.0	20
pCO_2 (kPa)	2.0	4.7 6

Q 12. What type of acid–base abnormality is shown? *1 mark*

Q 13. Explain how the low pCO_2 has occurred. *2 marks*

189

A venous blood sample sent for urea and electrolyte analysis gives the following results:

Parameter	Miss Winters' value (mmol/l)	Normal range (mmol/l)
Na	138	135–146
K	5.2	3.5–5.0
Cl	99	98–106
HCO$_3$	5.4	22–30
Urea	11.2	2.5–6.7
Creatinine	125	89–118

Q 14. What evidence is there that the patient is dehydrated?   *2 marks*

Q 15. Calculate the anion gap in this patient.   *1 mark*

Q 16. This anion gap is high. What is the normal gap?   *1 mark*

Q 17. Why has this large anion gap resulted in this patient?   *1 mark*

Whilst you are waiting for Miss Winters's blood results to return, you start treatment.

Q 18. Which aspect of Miss Winters's condition will you manage first
and how?
2 marks

Miss Winters's sister asks why their grandmother, who was only
diagnosed with diabetes last year, never has the same problem with
her illness that Miss Winters does.

Q 19. What endocrine emergency can occur in type II diabetics? *1 mark*

Q 20. This condition requires anticoagulation in addition to management of
the metabolic emergency. Which drug is used in this purpose? *1 mark*

📖 BIBLIOGRAPHY

Kumar P, Clark M. 2000. *Acute Clinical Medicine*. Sutton, Surrey: Reed Healthcare
Publishing.

Kumar P, Clark M. 2005. *Clinical Medicine,* 6th edn. Edinburgh: Elsevier Saunders.

McHardy K C, Godden D J, Nathwani D, Needham G, Duguid K P. 1994. *Illustrated
Cases in Acute Clinical Medicine*. Edinburgh: Churchill Livingstone.

Sawyer N, Gabriel R, Gabriel C M. 1989. *300 Medical Data Interpretation Questions
for MRCP*, 3rd edn. London: Butterworths.

ENDOCRINOLOGY

ENDOCRINOLOGY
3. THYROID DISEASE

You are a GP at the University Health Centre. Miss Taylor, a 19-year-old student, comes to see you complaining of having 'a lot of nervous energy'. In the past four months, she has been sweating excessively and has lost 5 kg despite having an increased appetite. She has also been having difficulty concentrating on her studies and is finding the lecture theatres too warm. You notice Miss Taylor has exophthalmos; the upper edge of both corneas being visible. She also has a tremor and her pulse is 102 beats per minute at rest.

You suspect that Miss Taylor has hyperthyroidism.

Q 1. What is the normal relationship of the upper lid to the cornea?   *1 mark*

Q 2. Name the thyroid hormones and indicate which is more potent.   *3 marks*

Q 3. One of the main actions of thyroid hormones is to regulate the basal metabolic rate (BMR). Define BMR.   *2 marks*

Q **4. The diagram below (Figure 7.5) shows a thyroid follicle. Label the parts indicated.** *2 marks*

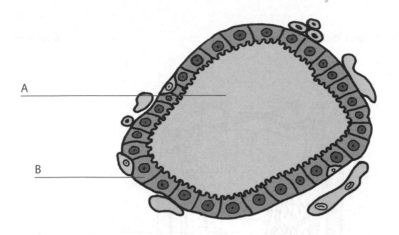

Figure 7.5: A thyroid follicle.

A – _____

B – _____

Q **5. Outline two functions of thyroid follicular cells.** *2 marks*

_____

_____

Q **6. Name the main protein that transports thyroid hormones in the plasma.** *1 mark*

_____

You palpate Miss Taylor's neck and discover that her thyroid gland is enlarged. It is smooth, non-tender and moves upwards with swallowing.

Q 7. **Label the diagram below (Figure 7.6).** *8 marks*

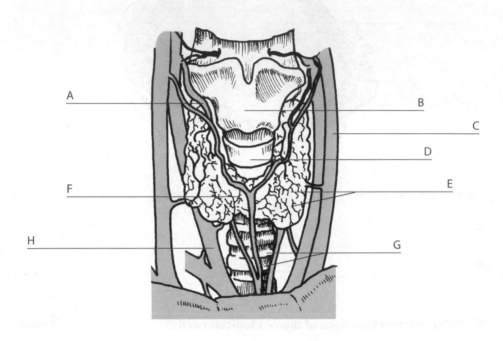

Figure 7.6: Thyroid anatomy.

A –

B –

C –

D –

E –

F – _____

G – _____

H – _____

Q 8. Why does the thyroid gland move upwards on swallowing?　　*1 mark*

_____

Miss Taylor asks you whether the thyroid enlargement is due to a deficiency in her diet.

Q 9. Name two components derived from the diet that are required for the synthesis of thyroid hormones.　　*1 mark*

_____

To confirm the diagnosis of hyperthyroidism, you take a blood sample from Miss Taylor and order thyroid function tests. To interpret the results you need to remember how thyroid hormones are regulated.

Q 10. Briefly describe the regulation of thyroid hormone secretion.　　*2 marks*

_____

_____

Q 11. What results would you expect from the thyroid function tests to confirm a diagnosis of primary hyperthyroidism?　　*1 mark*

_____

ENDOCRINOLOGY

The tests confirm primary hyperthyroidism and Miss Taylor is prescribed carbimazole. She takes the drug for 24 months but unfortunately experiences recurrent disease one year after stopping treatment. She does not want to take radio-iodine treatment and is referred for a surgical opinion. The surgeon recommends a subtotal thyroidectomy (ie partial removal of the thyroid gland) and explains the procedure and some of the complications that sometimes arise.

Q 12. Name the nerves that must be spared during neck surgery to ensure that no voice hoarseness occurs post-operatively. *2 marks*

The surgeon is careful to preserve the parathyroid glands.

Q 13. How many parathyroid glands are there and why are they at risk? *2 marks*

Q 14. What is the effect of a fall in parathyroid hormone levels (a) on blood calcium and (b) on bone? *2 marks*

Miss Taylor was successfully treated with partial thyroidectomy and has experienced no recurrence in her disease. She is concentrating better on her studies and is currently working towards her final exams. However, she is occasionally anxious that her symptoms may return since there is a 5% risk of relapse following surgery.

ENDOCRINOLOGY

📖 BIBLIOGRAPHY

Ellis H, Calne R, Watson C. 2006. *Lecture Notes. General Surgery*, 11th edn. London: Blackwell Publishing.

Franklyn J A. 1993. Hyperthyroidism. *Med Int*, **21**, 164–169.

Ganong W F. 2005. *Review of Medical Physiology*, 22nd edn. New York: McGraw-Hill Medical.

Kumar P, Clark M. 2005. *Clinical Medicine*, 6th edn. Edinburgh: Elsevier Saunders.

Tortora G J, Grabowski S R. 2000. *Principles of Anatomy and Physiology*, 9th edn. New York: John Wiley and Sons.

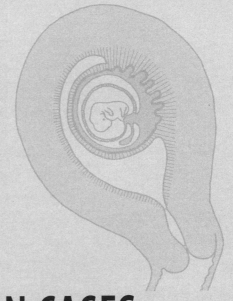

REPRODUCTION CASES: QUESTIONS

REPRODUCTION
1. FERTILITY

You are a GP registrar in the middle of a general surgery one afternoon. Your next appointment is for a Mrs Young whom you have not met before. You have a quick look through her medical notes before calling her through. You note that Mrs Young has a repeat prescription for the combined oral contraceptive pill.

Q 1. What is a 'combined oral contraceptive pill'?   *1 mark*

Q 2. Describe the three major actions of the combined oral
contraceptive pill.   *3 marks*

Mrs Young has not requested her oral contraceptive prescription for a number of months. You wonder if she is here about a pregnancy.

Q 3. Describe the sequence of events that occurs in the ovary during the
menstrual cycle under the following headings.   *5 marks*

Follicular phase (3 marks).

Ovulation (1 mark).

Luteal phase (1 mark).

Q 4. The following terms describe features of the ovarian follicles.
      Define each of the terms.   *3 marks*

4(a). Follicular atresia (1 mark).

4(b). Secondary follicle (1 mark).

4(c). Zona pellucida (1 mark).

Q 5. During a normal menstrual cycle, through which three phases
      does the endometrium pass and on which days of the cycle do they
      occur?   *3 marks*

Endometrial phase	Days of menstrual cycle

1 mark for being able to name each phase and the corresponding days of the
cycle; 3 marks in total.

Mrs Young comes into your surgery looking anxious. Her news is
not what you expect. She tells you that she and her husband have
been trying unsuccessfully to conceive for the last six months.
She is particularly concerned about her husband's fertility as he
suffered from mumps when he was 17.

Q 6. What is mumps and what organs does it affect?   *3 marks*

_____

_____

_____

Q 7. Identify A–J on the following diagram (Figure 8.1) of the male reproductive tract.   *5 marks*

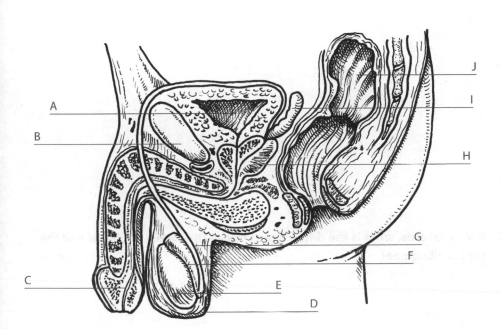

A
B
C
D
E
F
G
H
I
J

Figure 8.1: The male reproductive tract.

½ mark for each of the following:

A –

B –

C –

D –

E –

F –

G –

H –

I –

J –

Q 8. At the testis, what is the difference between the tunica vaginalis and the tunica albuginea?   *2 marks*

Q 9. What two cell populations are found in the seminiferous tubules of the testes?   *1 mark*

Q 10. Place the following in order of development. *1 mark*

- **Spermatocyte**
- **Spermatogonium**
- **Spermatid**
- **Spermatozoon**

Q 11. At which of the above stages is the chromosome number halved by meiosis? *1 mark*

Q 12. What is the function of the interstitial (Leydig[a]) cells of the testes and what controls their function? *1 mark*

Mrs Young asks how to go about having her husband's fertility checked and wonders about a semen sample.

Q 13. What term is used when there are fewer than 10 million spermatozoa per millilitre? *1 mark*

You explain to Mrs Young that male infertility is a rare complication of mumps but that you would be happy to see her husband to allay any concerns. You advise, however, that fertility tests are stressful and that the majority of patients conceive within a year of regular unprotected sexual intercourse. Mrs Young decides to wait until this time before commencing investigations.

REPRODUCTION

📖 BIBLIOGRAPHY

Fawcett D W. 1994. *A Textbook of Histology*. New York: Chapman and Hall.

Glasier A, Gebbie A. 2000. *Handbook of Family Planning and Reproductive Healthcare*, 4th edn. London: Churchill Livingstone.

Monga A, Campbell S. 2006. *Gynaecology by Ten Teachers*, 18th edn. London: Hodder Arnold.

Sadler T W. 2006. *Langman's Essential Medical Embryology*, 10th edn. London: Lippincott, Williams and Wilkins.

Tortora G J, Grabowski S R. *Principles of Anatomy and Physiology*, 10th edn. New York: John Wiley & Sons.

[a]Franz von Leydig (1821–1908), German zoologist and comparative anatomist who discovered the interstitial cells of the testis in 1850. He also defined cell types in the epidermis of fish and amphibians and in connective tissue and blood vessels of crustaceans.

REPRODUCTION
2. PREGNANCY

Two months after her first consultation Mrs Young is once again (see Case 1, Fertility) one of the patients in your afternoon general surgery. This time she looks much happier. She tells you that she thinks she is pregnant as her period is three weeks late and she has had a positive result on a home pregnancy test.

Q 1. Explain how the ELISA (enzyme-linked immunosorbent assay) home pregnancy test works.   *2 marks*

Q 2. When is human chorionic gonadotropin first detectable in the pregnant woman's urine?   *1 mark*

Q 3. In the first three months of pregnancy, which tissue produces human chorionic gonadotropin?   *1 mark*

Q 4. What is the action of human chorionic gonadotropin on the ovary?   *1 mark*

Q 5. In the second and third trimesters, what is the main source of progesterone?

1 mark

Q 6. Name two actions of progesterone during pregnancy.

1 mark

Having confirmed Mrs Young's pregnancy you offer her your congratulations as she is obviously very pleased. You ask her the date of the first day of her last period and confirm that she has a regular 28-day menstrual cycle. From this information you estimate that she is about 5 weeks pregnant.

Q 7. Identify A–F on this diagram (Figure 8.2) of the early pregnant uterus.

6 marks

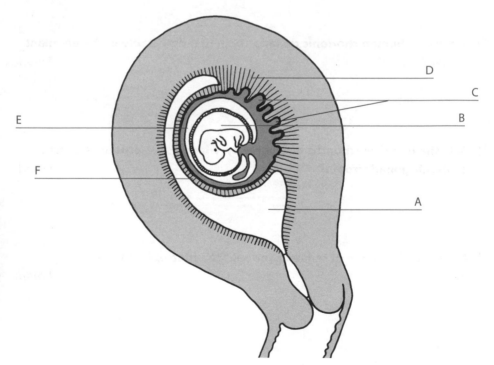

Figure 8.2: The early pregnant uterus.

½ mark for each of the following:

A –

B –

C –

D –

E –

F –

Q 8. When does the pregnant uterus first become palpable on
abdominal examination?   *1 mark*

Q 9. Name the tissues found in a placental villus at 3 months of
pregnancy.   *2 marks*

Q 10. Which tissues form the placental barrier at its thinnest part from
the 4th month of pregnancy onwards?   *1 mark*

Q 11. What is meant by the term 'syncytial knot'?   *1 mark*

Q 12. Define the following terms. *3 marks*

12(a). Placental cotyledon.

12(b). Placenta praevia.

12(c). Battledore placenta.

You establish that Mrs Young is still taking the folic acid you advised before conception and reiterate the importance of continuing with this supplement for the first three months of pregnancy to help prevent neural tube defects.

Q 13. What are the three embryonic germ layers? *1½ marks*

Q 14. Describe the four major stages in the formation of the neural tube. *2 marks*

Q 15. Explain the importance of folate in the prevention of neural tube defects. *1½ marks*

You measure Mrs Young's blood pressure and note that it is relatively low at 102/64 mmHg. You explain that women often have a drop in blood pressure during the first few months of pregnancy.

Q 16. Give two other ways in which the maternal cardiovascular system
adapts to pregnancy.   *2 marks*

You see from Mrs Young's medical notes that she is blood group O
Rhesus negative. You explain to Mrs Young the significance of this
for her pregnancy and ask if she knows whether her husband is
Rhesus negative or positive. Mrs Young agrees to find out.

Q 17. Explain the significance of a Rhesus negative blood group in a first
pregnancy.   *2 marks*

📖 BIBLIOGRAPHY

Baker P N. 2006. *Obstetrics by Ten Teachers*, 18th edn. London: Hodder Arnold.

Sadler T W. 2006. *Langman's Essential Medical Embryology*, 10th edn. London:
Lippincott, Williams and Wilkins.

Standring S. 2005. *Gray's Anatomy*, 39th edn. Edinburgh: Elsevier Churchill
Livingstone.

REPRODUCTION

REPRODUCTION
3. PROSTATE

You are the registrar at the urology clinic. One of the patients is Mr Grierson who has been referred by his GP. Mr Grierson is 61 years old. He had been asked to attend the well-man clinic at his GP's surgery and made up his mind it was the opportunity to see the doctor about his prostate problems. His 66-year-old brother, Robert, is being treated for cancer of the prostate and in recent months Mr Grierson has been having to get up through the night to pass urine. He has also been noticing that on voiding urine it is difficult to get the stream started. Mr Grierson has been otherwise well but knows that these are signs of prostatic disease but had been putting off seeking help.

Q 1. Label the following on the diagram (Figure 8.3):
- Anal canal
- Bulb of penis
- Bulbospongiosus muscle
- Corpus cavernosum
- Corpus spongiosum
- Ductus (vas) deferens
- Ejaculatory duct
- Neck of bladder
- Prostate
- Urethral sphincter

(½ mark for each, 5 marks in total)

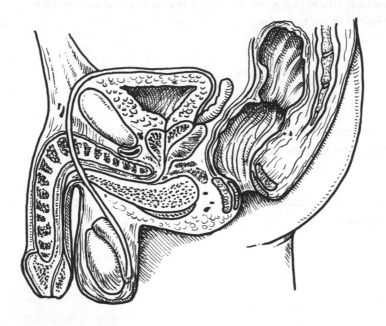

Figure 8.3: Male reproductive tract.

The sensation of needing to pass urine comes from stretch receptors in the wall of the urinary bladder as it comes under tension.

Q **2. To which segments of the spinal cord do primary sensory neurons pass from the bladder?** *1 mark*

Having listened to the history you take a blood sample for analysis of urea and electrolytes and for prostate-specific antigen.

Q **3. What is prostate-specific antigen?** *1 mark*

Q 4. Give four situations in which serum levels of prostate-specific antigen are likely to be raised.   *2 marks*

You carry out a rectal examination to check for prostatic hypertrophy or prostatic cancer.

Q 5. How would you distinguish these two conditions at rectal examination?   *2 mark*

Q 6. What is the rectovesical pouch and is it palpable at rectal examination?   *3 marks*

At rectal examination, you palpate a symmetrical diffuse enlargement of rubbery consistency. A longitudinal groove is palpable in the midline and the rectal mucosa moves freely relative to the prostate.

Q 7. Are these abnormal features?   *2 marks*

Q 8. Why are urea and electrolytes checked?   *1 mark*

The urea and electrolytes prove to be in the normal range and the prostate-specific antigen levels show borderline elevation. The diagnosis is benign prostatic hypertrophy.

Q 9. Does the fact that Mr Grierson's brother has prostatic cancer increase his risk of developing the disease?   *1 mark*

Arrangements are made for Mr Grierson to have a transurethral resection of his prostate. Mr Grierson is a very well-informed man with a sharp mind and wants to know about the procedure and the possible risks of the surgery, especially with regard to urinary continence and sexual function.

Q 10. From the bladder outwards, what are the parts of the male urethra and what are the approximate lengths of each part?   *3 marks*

Q 11. The urethral (external) sphincter is the main muscle controlling continence of urine. Which part of the urethra does it surround? What is its nerve supply?   *2 marks*

Q 12. Which muscle helps expel the last drops of urine? *1 mark*

Q 13. Which nerves innervate the blood vessels of the corpora cavernosa or spongiosum and are responsible for initiating erection? *1 mark*

Q 14. In a healthy subject what prevents the ejaculate from entering the urinary bladder? *1 mark*

The transurethral resection of the prostate is carried out under general anaesthetic. Samples of prostatic tissue are sent for pathology to exclude carcinoma.

Q 15. Briefly describe the appearance of prostate tissue on light microscopy. *1 mark*

Q 16. What are amyloid bodies? *1 mark*

Q 17. What type of nerve fibre innervates the smooth muscle of the prostate that contracts at ejaculation? *1 mark*

In the first two days after surgery, Mr Grierson is alarmed by the presence of blood clots in his urine.

REPRODUCTION

Q 18. What is the likely source of these blood clots? *1 mark*

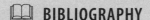 **BIBLIOGRAPHY**

http://www.cancer.org/docroot/CRI/content/CRI_2_4_3X_Can_prostate_cancer_be_found_early_36.asp

Browse N L. 1991. *An Introduction to the Symptoms and Signs of Surgical Disease*, 2nd edn. London: Edward Arnold.

Kumar P, Clark M. 2005. *Clinical Medicine*, 6th edn. Edinburgh: Elsevier Saunders.

Sinnatamby C S. 1999. *Last's Anatomy: Regional and Applied*, 10th edn. Edinburgh: Churchill Livingstone.

Standring S. 2005. *Gray's Anatomy*, 39th edn. Edinburgh: Elsevier Churchill Livingstone.

Steinberg G D, Carter B S, Beaty T H, Childs B, Walsh P C. 1990. Family history and the risk of prostate cancer. *Prostate*, **17**, 337–47.

Tortora G J, Grabowski S R. *Principles of Anatomy and Physiology*, 10th edn. New York: John Wiley & Sons.

Q. 16. What is the likely source of these wood dust?   1 mark

BIBLIOGRAPHY

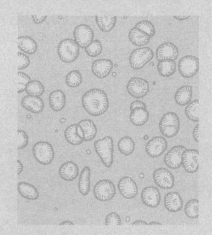

HAEMATOLOGY CASES:
QUESTIONS

HAEMATOLOGY
1. CHRONIC LYMPHOCYTIC LEUKAEMIA

You are a GP registrar called to the local residential home to assess Mr Burns, a 79-year-old man who has not been feeling well of late. His daughter has become increasingly worried about her father's well being. He is tired and breathless and has multiple unexplained bruises, particularly on his lower limbs.

On examination you discover he has hepatosplenomegaly and has evidence of bleeding into his oral mucosa.

Q 1. In a healthy adult, in which region of the abdominal cavity does the spleen normally lie?   *1 mark*

Q 2. At the level of which ribs does the spleen lie?   *1 mark*

Q 3. List four structures that lie between the spleen and the lower left ribs.   *2 marks*

Q 4. Through which fold of peritoneum does the splenic artery pass to reach the spleen?   *1 mark*

HAEMATOLOGY

Q 5. On the following CT of the upper abdomen (Figure 9.1), identify A–J. *5 marks*

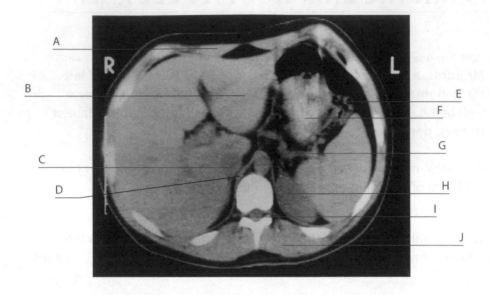

Figure 9.1: CT of the upper abdomen.

½ mark for each of the following:

A –

B –

C –

D –

E –

F –

G – _____

H – _____

I – _____

J – _____

The spleen is composed of red pulp and white pulp.

Q 6. Complete the table below indicating whether the features listed belong to the red or white pulp.   *3 marks*

½ mark for each correct answer

Feature	Red pulp or white pulp?
Aggregates of lymphocytes	
Splenic cords	
Splenic sinusoids	
Central arterioles	
Lymphoid nodules	
Penicillar arteries	

Q 7. Give four functions of the adult human spleen.   *2 marks*

Mr Burns is found to be anaemic, with a high white cell count, and his platelets are extremely low (thrombocytopaenia). Differential white cell count shows a lymphocytosis.

The haematologist takes charge of Mr Burns's management and admits him to hospital for further investigations. She carries out a bone marrow trephine and aspirate.

Q 8. From which anatomical site are these samples most likely to be taken?   *1 mark*

Q 9. For what purpose is: (a) a trephine sample and (b) an aspirate sample collected?   *2 marks*

A diagnosis of chronic lymphocytic leukaemia is made and Mr Burns is transferred to a side room, as he is vulnerable to infection.

Q 10. Explain why Mr Burns is vulnerable to infection.   *1 mark*

Q 11. Why is he anaemic and thrombocytopaenic?   *1 mark*

Q 12. Which cell type is responsible for the production of platelets?   *1 mark*

Q 13. Complete this flow diagram (Figure 9.2) showing the different cell lines that occur in haemopoiesis.   *4 marks*

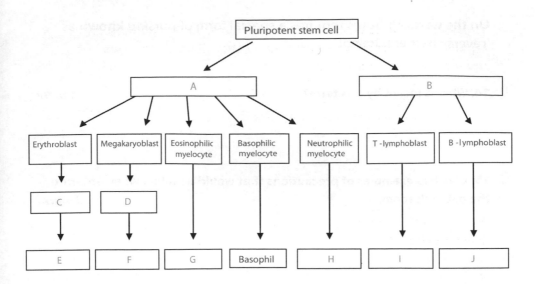

Figure 9.2: Haemopoiesis.

1/3 mark for each:

A –

B –

C –

D –

E –

F –

G –

H –

I –

J –

On the ward, Mr Burns requires a special form of nursing known as 'reverse barrier nursing'.

Q 14. What is meant by this term?   *1 mark*

Q 15. Give two examples of precautions that would be taken when entering the patient's room.   *2 marks*

As part of his treatment, Mr Burns requires a blood transfusion.

Blood used for transfusion is collected from donors and is processed into different blood components and products.

Q 16. Name two blood components and two blood products.   *2 marks*

📖 BIBLIOGRAPHY

Abrahams P, Craven J, Lumley J. 2005. *Illustrated Clinical Anatomy*. London: Hodder Arnold.

Kumar P, Clark M. 2005. *Clinical Medicine*, 6th edn. Edinburgh: Elsevier Saunders.

Provan D, Krentz A. 2002. *Oxford Handbook of Clinical and Laboratory Investigation*. Oxford: Oxford University Press.

Sanders S, Dawson J, Datta S, Eccles S. 2005. *Oxford Handbook for the Foundation Programme*. Oxford: Oxford University Press.

Stevens A, Lowe J S. 2005. *Human Histology*, 3rd edn. Philadelphia: Elsevier Mosby.

Tortora G J, Derrickson B. 2006. *Principles of Anatomy and Physiology*, 11th edn. Hoboken, New Jersey: Wiley.

HAEMATOLOGY
2. IRON DEFICIENCY ANAEMIA

You are a final year medical student attached to a general practice. A 42-year-old woman, Mrs Forbes, comes to the surgery because she becomes tired easily when doing any physical work, even of a minor nature. The GP asks you to take a history from the patient. After asking a series of questions, you are surprised to find the patient has had heavy periods for the past year but has never sought medical help. You suspect iron deficiency anaemia due to chronic blood loss from menorrhagia. On examination Mrs Forbes has angular stomatitis and a smooth tongue.

Q 1. Define the term anaemia.   *1 mark*

You remember the production of red blood cells (erythropoiesis) requires certain essential micronutrients and hormonal factors.

Q 2. Name two micronutrients, apart from iron, that are essential in erythropoiesis.
2 marks

You know that erythropoietin (EPO) is the principal hormone regulating the process of erythropoiesis.

Q 3. What is the major site of erythropoietin production in a healthy adult?
1 mark

HAEMATOLOGY

Q 4. What is the major stimulus for its production?   *1 mark*

Red cell production and maturation take place in bone marrow and peripheral blood.

Q 5. The flow chart below (Figure 9.3) shows the process of erythropoiesis. Name A, B and C.   *3 marks*

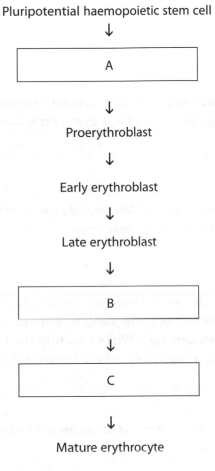

Pluripotential haemopoietic stem cell
↓

A

↓
Proerythroblast
↓
Early erythroblast
↓
Late erythroblast
↓

B

↓

C

↓
Mature erythrocyte

Figure 9.3: Erythropoiesis.

A –

B –

C –

Q 6. Name the erythrocyte precursor cell in which each of the following events/features are observed:

Q 6(a). Extrusion of the nucleus. *1 mark*

Q 6(b). The last erythrocyte precursor to contain ribosomes that, on staining for light microscopy, give a blue tinge to the cytoplasm. *1 mark*

Q 6(c). The erythrocyte precursor that may appear in increased numbers in the peripheral blood following blood loss. *1 mark*

The GP takes a blood sample from Mrs Forbes for full blood count and iron status, the working diagnosis being iron deficiency anaemia due to menorrhagia. While awaiting the result the GP asks you what you expect the results of the blood test will be if this is correct.

Q 7. Fill in the table below, indicating the expected results as increased, decreased or normal. *3 marks*

Parameter	Result
Haemoglobin	
Mean cell volume (MCV)	
Mean cell haemoglobin concentration (MCHC)	
Serum iron	
Total iron binding capacity (TIBC)	
Serum ferritin	

The film below is that of the patient (Figure 9.4).

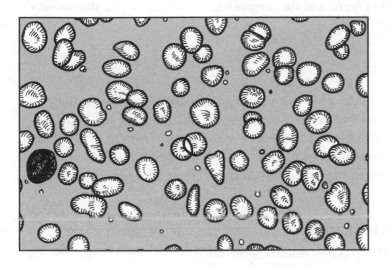

Figure 9.4: Blood film.

Q 8. Give two features of the blood film that indicate iron deficiency anaemia. *2 marks*

_____

_____

The white blood cell to the left of the microscope field has a diameter similar to that of healthy erythrocytes.

Q 9. What is this cell? *1 mark*

Q 10. Name one other formed element of blood visible in the drawing. *1 mark*

Q 11. In patients such as Mrs Forbes with glossitis due to iron deficiency anaemia, what feature of the tongue has atrophied to give the smooth appearance? *1 mark*

The GP also takes a full gynaecological history from the patient as she has had heavy menstrual periods for the past one year. Abdominal examination reveals a mass arising from the pelvis. Your GP refers the patient to the gynaecological department for further investigation. In the meantime, Mrs Forbes is prescribed ferrous sulphate.

One month later, Mrs Forbes returns to your GP surgery. The iron tablets have been making her constipated. The main reason for her current visit, however, is a problem with swallowing, particularly with solid foods.

Q 12. Label the parts shown in the figure below (Figure 9.5). *6 marks*

½ mark for each

A –

B –

C –

D –

E –

F –

G –

H –

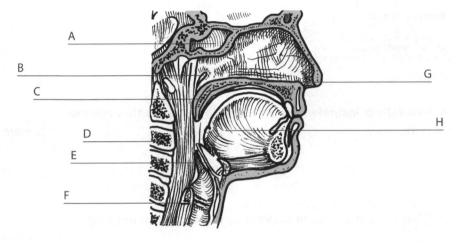

Figure 9.5: Throat anatomy.

In swallowing, reflexes move the bolus through the pharynx.

Q **13. Which muscle of the tongue moves the tongue backwards and upwards (posterosuperiorly)?** *1 mark*

Q 14. Which cranial nerve provides most of the sensory innervation of the oropharynx? *1 mark*

Q 15. Indicate which of the following phases of swallowing are voluntary and which are involuntary? *1½ marks*

Phase	Type of movement	Marks
Oral phase		½
Pharyngeal phase		½
Oesophageal phase		½

Q 16. Name the principal muscles that move the bolus through the pharynx. *½ mark*

Q 17. What is the main factor preventing food from entering the larynx? *1 mark*

The GP is concerned that Mrs Forbes may have chronic pharyngo-oesophagitis (Paterson–Brown–Kelly[a] disease/Plummer Vinson[b] syndrome), a condition associated with iron deficiency anaemia, and refers her to the ear, nose and throat department for further assessment.

The GP sees Mrs Forbes a month later. It had been a uterine fibroid that had been causing the heavy periods. Her problem swallowing is now improving with the iron tablets and she is about to see the otorhinolaryngologist.

📖 BIBLIOGRAPHY

Gray R F, Hawthorne M. 1992. *Synopsis of Otolaryngology*, 5th edn. Oxford: Butterworth Heinemann.

[a]D. R. Paterson (1863–1939) and A. Brown-Kelly (1865–1941), British surgeons who described sideropenic dysphagia independently in 1919.

[b]H. S. Plummer (1874–1936) and P. P. Vinson (1890–1959), American physicians from the Mayo Clinic, Minnesota, who also described the condition in 1912 and 1919 respectively – and whose names are used for its description within the USA.

HAEMATOLOGY
3. LYMPH NODES/HIV

You are the GP on duty one afternoon when a 33-year-old patient, Mr Reading, comes to see you because of swellings in his neck and armpits. He has been aware of these for the last four months and has also been feeling tired. He has no previous history of ill health.

After a thorough physical examination, you find that Mr Reading has enlarged lymph nodes, some greater than 2 cm, regular in contour, firm, mobile and non-tender on both sides in his axilla, neck and groin. He also has splenomegaly.

Q 1. List four lymphoid organs or tissues found in humans, apart from lymph nodes.   *2 marks*

Most of the lymphoid organs have an internal skeleton of reticular fibres.

Q 2. In brief, what is the composition of reticular fibres?   *1 mark*

Q 3. Give two principal functions of a lymph node.   *2 marks*

Q A diagram of the structure of a lymph node is shown below (Figure 9.6).

Q 4. Identify features A–H (Figure 9.6). *4 marks*

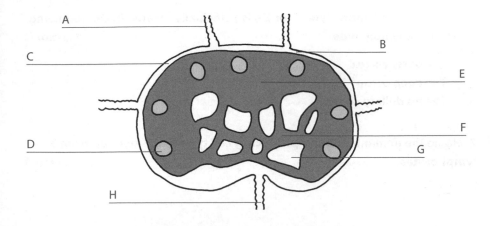

Figure 9.6: The structure of a lymph node.

½ mark for each:

A –

B –

C –

D –

E –

F –

G –

H –

Q 5. Why are T-lymphocytes called "T"-lymphocytes? *1 mark*

Q 6. Which type of lymphocyte, T- or B-, is principally located in the following regions of a lymph node? *1½ marks*

- The outer cortex
- The deep cortex
- The medullary cords?

Q 7. Name the immunoglobulin-producing cell type that is derived from B-lymphocytes. *½ mark*

On looking at his past notes you see that Mr Reading is a recovered heroin addict who was using intravenous drugs for three years before entering a rehabilitation programme. He has now been free of drug abuse for 1 year.

In view of Mr Reading's history you feel that a human immune deficiency virus (HIV) test would be appropriate. He consents to this and admits that the possibility of HIV had been worrying him for some time.

Q 8. What type of virus is HIV? *1 mark*

Q 9. Which enzyme is used by viruses such as HIV to form DNA for inclusion in the host genome? *1 mark*

Q 10. A drawing of this virus is shown below (Figure 9.7). Please name the indicated features. *2 marks*

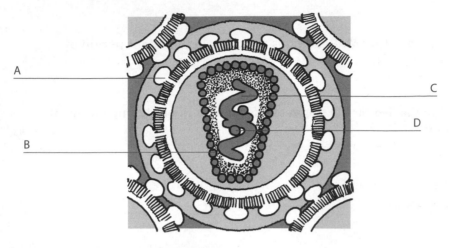

Figure 9.7: The human immunodeficiency virus.

Features labelled (½ mark for each):

A –

B –

C –

D –

Q 11. Outline six main steps involved in replication of HIV in vivo. *3 marks*

Q 12. Name the specific cell type which is reduced in HIV infection. *1 mark*

You believe that Mr Reading is probably in the latent period of infection.

Q 13. List the five clinical stages of infection for HIV including the latent period. *4 marks*

Q 14. Give three modes of transmission of HIV. *1 mark*

Mr Reading wishes to know about treatment. Although there is no current treatment to completely eradicate infection, there are drugs that can suppress the virus even below limits of detection. You tell him that anti-retroviral drugs are the main method of treatment.

Q 15. Explain how these drugs work. *2 marks*

Q 16. What tests could you do to monitor Mr Reading's progress? *1 mark*

Q 17. Give two other pieces of advice you would like to tell Mr Reading.   *1 mark*

Q 18. Finally, name the primary opportunistic infection seen in HIV disease.   *1 mark*

📖 BIBLIOGRAPHY

Boon NA, Colledge NR, Walker BR, Hunter JAA. 2006. *Davidson's Principles and Practice of Medicine*, 20th edn. Edinburgh: Elsevier Churchill Livingstone.

British National Formulary – September 2004. London: British Medical Association, Royal Pharmaceutical Society of Great Britain.

Kumar P, Clark M. 1998. *Clinical Medicine*. London: WB Saunders.

Longmore M, Wilkinson I, Turmezei T, Cheung CK, Smith E. 2007. *Oxford Handbook of Clinical Medicine,* 7th edn. Oxford: Oxford University Press.

Mims C, Dockrell M, Goering R, Roitt I, Wakelin D, Zuckerman M. 2004. *Medical Microbiology*, 3rd edn. London: Mosby.

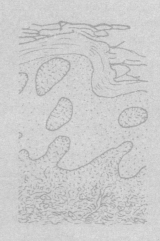

DERMATOLOGY CASE:
QUESTIONS

DERMATOLOGY
1. PSORIASIS

You are on duty in general practice one morning. The next patient to arrive is Miss Smith, an anxious 15-year-old girl who has come along to see you with her mother. She is embarrassed, as recently she has noticed skin changes particularly on her arms and around her knees.

On examination, you notice that there are numerous small round red plaques, with obvious scaling, present on her forearms, elbows, knees and shins. You make the diagnosis of psoriasis.

Q **1. What form of psoriasis is this most likely to be?** *1 mark*

Q **2. Describe *four* characteristic histological features of the skin in this disease.** *4 marks*

Below is a diagram showing the histology of psoriasis.

Q 3. Label normal skin structures A–D   *2 marks*

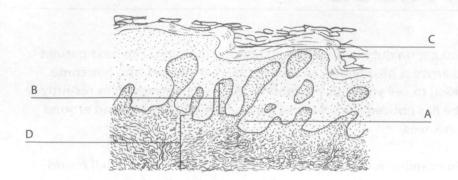

Figure 10.1: Skin structure.

A –

B –

C –

D –

Q 4. To what class of epithelium does epidermis belong?   *1 mark*

The normal epidermis is 50–150 μm thick.

Q 5. How much thicker can epidermis be in psoriasis, when compared with healthy skin?   *1 mark*

Keratinocytes are the main type of cell found in skin (~85%). These are held together by different types of intercellular contacts.

Q 6. Complete the table, giving the function of the following intercellular junctions (not specific to skin). *2 marks*

Name of junction	Function
Tight junction	
Gap junction	
Desmosome	
Hemidesmosome	

Q 7. State *four* changes which happen to keratinocytes as they mature and become differentiated. *2 marks*

As well as keratinocytes, three other cell types are found in the epidermis – melanocytes, Langerhans cells[a] and Merkel cells[b].

Q 8. In which skin layers are melanocytes found? *1 mark*

Q 9. Describe the appearance of a Langerhans cell. *2 marks*

Langerhans cells play an important role in the immune system.

Q 10. Outline *three* properties that they possess that allow them to present antigens effectively. *3 marks*

One feature of psoriasis is the Koebner phenomenon.

Q 11. What is this? *1 mark*

Q 12. Name *two* other conditions in which it occurs. *2 marks*

In psoriasis, pin-point bleeding can occur if a scale is scraped off (Auspitz sign)

Q 13. Why does this occur? *1 mark*

You go on to examine Miss Smith's nails as you are aware that there is an association between psoriasis and nail changes.

Q 14. What are nails made of and from where are they derived? *1 mark*

Q 15. Name *two* features of psoriatic nail involvement. *1 mark*

One form of psoriasis, guttate psoriasis, can be precipitated by a throat infection.

Q 16. What organism is responsible in this case? *1 mark*

At the end of the consultation you advise Miss Smith and her mother about treatment. If the condition does not remit spontaneously then vitamin D analogues are a treatment option.

Q 17. How do they work? *1 mark*

Q 18. Complete this table. *3 marks*

An example of vitamin D analogue	Advantages of vitamin D analogues (give 2)	Disadvantages of vitamin D analogues (give 2)

DERMATOLOGY

📖 BIBLIOGRAPHY

Hunter J A A, Savin J A, Dahl M V. 2002. *Clinical Dermatology*, 3rd edn. Oxford: Blackwell Science.

Kumar P, Clark M. 2005. *Clinical Medicine*, 6th edn. Edinburgh: Elsevier Saunders.

Longmore M, Wilkinson I, Turmezei T, Cheung CK, Smith E. 2007. *Oxford Handbook of Clinical Medicine*, 7th edn. Oxford: Oxford University Press.

MacKie R M. 2003. *Clinical Dermatology*, 5th edn. Oxford: Oxford University Press.

McPhee S J, Ganong W F. 2006. *Pathophysiology of Disease*, 5th edn. New York: Lange Medical Books/McGraw-Hill.

[a]Paul Langerhans (see page 483).

[b]Friedrich Sigmund Merkel (1845–1919), German anatomist and histopathologist who described 'Tastzellum' (touch cells) in the skin of vertebrates.

ANSWERS

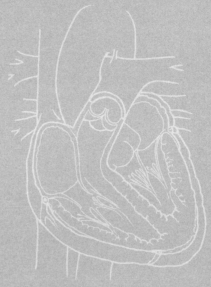

CARDIOLOGY CASES:
ANSWERS

CARDIOLOGY
1. CONGENITAL HEART DISEASE

You are a junior doctor working in the Paediatric Accident and Emergency Department. Mrs Smith, a 32-year-old mother, presents with her 6-week-old baby, Jack. Mrs Smith says Jack has been sweating and increasingly breathless during his feeds over the past week or so. He has also been quite irritable over this period. Prior to this, Baby Jack was well and he was on the 50th centile for head circumference, length and weight. His neonatal examination was normal.

You examine Jack, and note he is tachypnoeic (60 breaths per minute), and tachycardic (170 beats per minute). He is not cyanosed, and there are no signs of upper airway obstruction, though there is slight wheeze and intercostal recession.

You auscultate Jack's precordium, listening for heart sounds and murmurs. You hear a loud pansystolic murmur at the lower left sternal edge with a split second heart sound. On listening to the chest, you hear scattered wheezes. From the history and examination, you suspect a congenital heart defect and arrange an ECG, chest X-ray and echocardiogram.

📁 **LEARNING POINT**

Congenital heart defects

Congenital heart defects (CHDs) occur in around 8 per 1000 births. Some defects are caused by single-gene or chromosomal abnormalities, while others arise from exposure to teratogens (eg Rubella virus). Most defects, however, arise from a combination of genetic and environmental factors.

As you wait for the above investigations to be carried out, you revise the anatomy and physiology of the fetal circulation.

Q **1. Label the following diagram of the fetal circulation.** *4 marks*

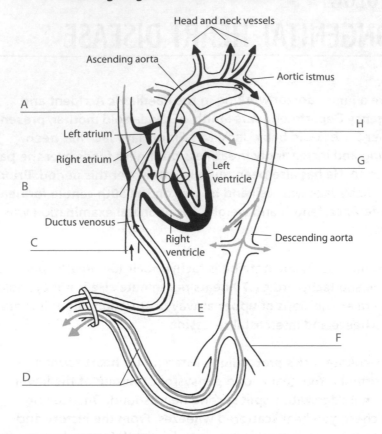

Figure 1.1: Anatomy of fetal circulation.

A ½ mark each:

   A – Superior vena cava

   B – Foramen ovale

   C – Inferior vena cava

   D – Umbilical arteries

   E – Umbilical vein

   F – Left common iliac artery

   G – Pulmonary trunk

   H – Ductus arteriosus

Q 2. Please answer the following questions on the fetal circulation. *4 marks*

Q 2(a). Through which opening does deoxygenated blood leave the fetal right atrium?

A Tricuspid valve (1 mark).

Q 2(b). In which organ does the ductus venosus lie?

A Liver (1 mark).

Q 2(c). What does the umbilical vein become after birth?

A The round ligament of the liver (ligamentum teres) (1 mark).

Q 2(d). Which atrium of the heart, left or right, has the higher pressure in its chamber during fetal life?

A Right (1 mark).

You consider the development of the fetal heart, which initially forms as a tubular structure and is subsequently partitioned.

Q 3. At what age does the early heart begin to beat? *1 mark*

A 21–23 days.

Please look at the following diagram of the early heart.

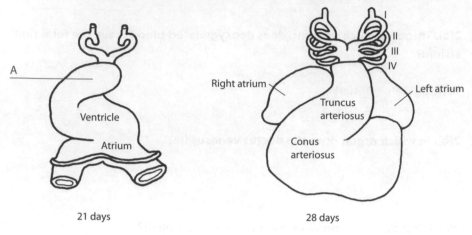

Figure 1.2: Anatomy of the early heart.

Q 4. Structure A is the outflow tract in the early embryonic heart. What is this structure commonly called? *1 mark*

A Bulbus cordis.

Q 5. Which structures form from the truncus arteriosus, the distal part of structure A? *1 mark*

A Ascending aorta and pulmonary trunk (1 mark for both).

Q 6. Postganglionic sympathetic and parasympathetic neurons become associated with the developing heart. What is the embryological source of these ganglion cells? *1 mark*

A Neural crest.

Q 7. On the diagram of the fetal heart at 28 days, there are structures labelled I–IV. What are these structures collectively known as? *1 mark*

A Aortic arches or pharyngeal arch arteries.

📂 LEARNING POINT

Four aortic arch pairs are shown here. Six pairs develop in total, although the fifth pair is rudimentary. They are not all present simultaneously, however. By the time the sixth pair of aortic arches has formed, the first two pairs have usually regressed.

Q 8. Structures I–IV above eventually form various definitive structures. Name two such adult structures that are derived from I–IV. *1 mark*

A ½ mark each for any two of the following:

- Aortic arch

- Right subclavian artery

- Right and left common carotid arteries

📂 LEARNING POINT

The fetal aortic arches undergo complex changes before forming the adult arterial arrangement. Portions of the aortic arches may disappear or persist inappropriately, giving rise to anomalies. Examples of such anomalies include:
- Coarctation of the aorta
- Double aortic arch
- Right arch of the aorta
- Anomalous right subclavian artery

The echocardiography report for Baby Jack becomes available, and confirms a congenital heart lesion – a ventricular septal defect (VSD). You consider how Baby Jack's symptoms can be explained by this pathology.

Q 9. You first of all consider the normal pressures in the chambers of the adult heart. Please complete the following table of pressures within the chambers of the heart, using the options below. (Each option may be used once, more than once, or not at all.)   *4 marks*

- <10 mmHg
- 25 mmHg
- 40 mmHg
- 80 mmHg
- 120 mmHg
- 180 mmHg

Chamber of heart	Blood pressure (mmHg)	
	Systolic	Diastolic
Right atrium	< 10	< 10
Right ventricle	25	< 10
Left atrium	< 10	< 10
Left ventricle	120	< 10

A ½ mark for each.

You recall, however, that the equivalent blood pressures in the neonate and infant are much lower than the adult values shown above.

Q 10. In what direction is blood flowing across Baby Jack's VSD?   *1 mark*

A Left ventricle → Right ventricle.

Q 11. At which part of the interventricular septum does a congenital defect most commonly occur?   *1 mark*

A Membranous part of the interventricular septum.

📁 LEARNING POINT

The interventricular septum forms embryologically at the same time as the interatrial septum. A thick muscular ridge forms in the floor of the primitive ventricle near the apex of the heart. Differential muscular proliferation of the ventricular walls creates an enlarging septum. The right and left bulbar ridges form in the truncus arteriosus, meet each other and partition the truncus arteriosus to give the ascending aorta and the pulmonary trunk. The inferior edge of this partition meets the muscular part of the interventricular septum and the endocardial cushions, forming the atrioventricular valves, to complete the interventricular septum by forming its upper membranous part. By the end of the seventh week, the septum is complete. Defects in the formation of this small membranous part of the septum give the majority of interventricular septal defects.

You recall that on auscultating Jack's precordium, you heard a loud pansystolic murmur at the lower left sternal edge with a fixed, split second heart sound.

Q 12. In general, what can you can deduce about the size of a VSD if it produces a loud murmur? *1 mark*

A Loud murmurs are produced by smaller defects; quieter murmurs are produced by larger defects.

📁 LEARNING POINT

A smaller VSD opening will be associated with a greater pressure difference between the two sides of the opening. This causes more turbulent flow, and thus a louder murmur. If the VSD is very large, the rate of turbulent flow would be less, and this would create a quieter murmur. In very large VSDs, however, there tends to be a pulmonary ejection murmur from high volume flow across the pulmonary valve. Very large VSDs, therefore, tend to be associated with pulmonary murmurs.

Q 13. Explain why the murmur found in Baby Jack is pansystolic. *1 mark*

A Turbulent flow of blood occurs through the defect whenever the ventricles are contracting. The murmur is thus pansystolic.

Q 14. Explain why the fixed split second heart sound is produced in Baby Jack. *2 marks*

A ½ mark for each of the following:

- The VSD causes volume overload in the right side of the heart

- Right ventricular systole is longer in duration

- This results in delayed closure of the pulmonary valve compared to closure of the aortic valve

- The second heart sound is 'fixed' because inspiration and expiration make no significant difference to the end-diastolic volume of blood in the right ventricle. The right ventricle is, in this case, always volume overloaded, irrespective of respiratory movements

Q 15. With reference to fetal circulation and changes in the cardiovascular system that occur in the weeks after birth, why has Baby Jack been asymptomatic with his VSD up until now, 6 weeks after birth? Why is he symptomatic now? *2 marks*

A When the baby is born the pulmonary vascular resistance is still relatively high (1 mark) and the right ventricle relatively 'stronger' than it is later (1 mark), reflecting the fetal dynamics of the circulation to the placenta. An alternative answer is: The pulmonary vascular resistance falls in the weeks after birth as the lungs grow (1 mark) and develop a more extensive pulmonary vasculature. The left ventricle also hypertrophies over this time (1 mark).

Q 16. You look at Baby Jack's chest X-ray and note that the cardiothoracic ratio is around 55%. Is this abnormal? *1 mark*

A In an infant of 6 weeks, a cardiothoracic ratio of > 50% is physiologically normal (1 mark). This is not a cause for concern and is not necessarily a consequence of heart failure.

📁 LEARNING POINT

Cardiac size can be readily assessed on the PA chest X-ray, using the cardiothoracic ratio (CTR):

$$\text{Cardiothoracic ratio} = \frac{\text{Maximum transverse diameter of the heart}}{\text{Maximum transverse diameter of the thorax (inner aspect of ribs)}}$$

The CTR is usually less than 50% in healthy adults, with anything greater than 50% termed 'cardiomegaly'.

In neonates, infants and athletes, however, the heart is physiologically (ie not pathologically) larger, occupying a larger proportion of the thoracic diameter. The CTR is thus often >50%.

Individuals with skeletal abnormalities such as scoliosis may also have a CTR of more than 50%. This is likely to reflect a reduction in thoracic cavity diameter rather than an increase in cardiac dimensions

Q 17. Describe one other change you would expect to see on Baby Jack's chest X-ray. *1 mark*

A 1 mark for any of the following:

- Increased pulmonary vascular markings (alveolar oedema)

- Left atrial/left ventricular enlargement

- Upper lobe diversion/enlarged pulmonary arteries

You decide to treat Baby Jack with furosemide before referring him to the paediatric cardiologists for their opinion and possible surgery.

CARDIOLOGY

Q 18. With reference to cardiac workload, how would furosemide help with Baby Jack's symptoms? *2 marks*

- Furosemide causes venodilation (1 mark) (and some arteriolar vasodilatation) helping to reduce preload (and to an extent afterload).

- Furosemide, over the few hours after administration, also causes a diuresis helping to reduce circulating blood volume (1 mark). This also reduces preload.

A This allows both sides of the heart to pump with a greater cardiac output, reducing pulmonary congestion.

📖 BIBLIOGRAPHY

Barnes N, Archer N. 2005. Understanding congenital heart disease. *Current Paediatrics*, **15,** 421–428.

Brown K. 2005. The infant with undiagnosed cardiac disease in the emergency department. *Clinical Pediatric Emergency Medicine*, **6**, 200–206.

Carlson B M. 2004. *Human Embryology and Developmental Biology*, 3rd edn. New York: Elsevier, p. 447

Julian D G, Cowan J C, McLenachan J M. 2005. *Cardiology*, 8th edn. London: Elsevier Saunders.

Lissauer T, Clayden G. 2007. *Illustrated Textbook of Paediatrics*, 2nd edn. Edinburgh: Mosby.

Moore K L, Persaud T V N. 2003. *The Developing Human: Clinically Orientated Embryology*, 7th edn. London: Saunders.

Newby D E, Grubb N R. 2005. *Cardiology: An Illustrated Colour Text*. London: Churchill Livingstone, p. 134.

CARDIOLOGY
2. DOWN SYNDROME AND CONGENITAL CARDIAC ABNORMALITIES

You are on call in paediatrics, when you are asked to visit Baby Taylor, a newborn baby on the maternity ward, for a 'baby check' examination. While carrying out your examination you notice some dysmorphic features, and you think that Baby Taylor may have Down syndrome[a].

Q 1. List six dysmorphic features, visible on inspection, which are commonly associated with Down syndrome. *3 marks*

A Any six of the following (½ mark each)

Facial features:

- Round face
- Epicanthic folds/flat nasal bridge
- Protruding tongue
- Small ears

Other dysmorphic features:

- Single palmar creases (simian crease)
- Flat occiput
- Short or incurved little fingers (little fingers bent towards others)
- Gap between first and second toes (sandal toe gap)
- Small stature.

Q 2. Name one neurological finding which is likely to be found on examination of Baby Taylor. *1 mark*

A Hypotonia.

 LEARNING POINT

Neurological findings

Hypotonia is a common finding in children with Down syndrome. Developmental delay is also a neurological finding in Down syndrome; however, it is not an appropriate answer in this instance as the examination is of a newborn baby.

Q 3. What is the commonest genetic abnormality in Down syndrome? *1 mark*

A Trisomy 21.

 LEARNING POINT

Trisomy 21

Trisomy 21 is the most common autosomal trisomy compatible with life. There are three possible mechanisms of trisomy 21:

- **Non-disjunction:** (95%) pair of chromosomes 21 fails to separate at meiosis; 90% of these are maternally derived, the risk rising with maternal age
- **Translocation:** (4%) translocation of the third chromosome 21 onto another chromosome, most commonly 14 – the Robertsonian translocation. This is the cause of familial Down syndrome
- **Mosaicism:** (1%) the non-disjunction occurs during mitosis after formation of the zygote. This produces some normal cells and some trisomy 21 cells, often producing a milder phenotype

You discover that Mrs Taylor is aged 42 years with a possible family history of Down syndrome. She was offered antenatal diagnostic tests but declined.

Q **4. What test would she have been offered?** *1 mark*

A Testing of fetal chromosomes (½ mark), with fetal cells obtained by chorionic villus sampling (½ mark) or by amniocentesis (½ mark).

Q **5. Approximately how common is Down syndrome in pregnancies where the mother is over 40 years of age: 1 in 25; 1 in 100; 1 in 1000; 1 in 10 000?** *1 mark*

A 1 in 100.

You report your suspicions to your consultant, who agrees with your diagnosis. On examination of Baby Taylor he also hears a heart murmur. He informs Mr and Mrs Taylor that he suspects their child has Down syndrome and that he would like to arrange some genetic tests. He also explains that some children with Down syndrome are at a higher risk of other medical problems, and that he is also going to arrange some tests to look at Baby Taylor's heart.

📁 **LEARNING POINT**

Communicating with parents about the diagnosis of Down syndrome
- A senior paediatrician should always confirm suspicion about the diagnosis and inform the parents prior to genetic testing
- Parents should be informed of the diagnosis together if possible, or there should be a support network (friend or relative) in the case of a young or single parent
- Parents need information about the implications of the diagnosis and the assistance available from professionals and self-help groups
- Genetic counselling about future pregnancy will be required

Q **6. What is the most appropriate investigation to visualise Baby Taylor's heart and its function?** *1 mark*

A Doppler[b] (½ mark) echocardiogram (½ mark).

Q **7. Apart from cardiac abnormalities, name one other structural congenital abnormality commonly associated with Down syndrome.** *1 mark*

- Duodenal atresia (1 mark)

- Congenital cataracts (1 mark)

- Atlanto-axial subluxation (½ mark)

📁 LEARNING POINT

Structural abnormalities associated with Down syndrome

Many conditions occur with increased frequency in children with Down syndrome. Excluding the congenital cardiac abnormalities, which occur in approximately 40% of children with Down syndrome, duodenal atresia is by far the most common structural problem. It occurs in approximately 5% of those with the syndrome. Approximately one-third of children born with duodenal atresia have Down syndrome.

Other structural problems include
- **Congenital cataracts**
- **Osteoarticular problems. This is rare in the paediatric age group but occurs in approximately 15% of patients with Down syndrome at some stage in their lifetime. Most are asymptomatic and only 1%–2% require treatment**
- **Other GI conditions – oesophageal atresia, Meckel's diverticulum, umbilical hernia, Hirschprung's disease and imperforate anus. These, however, do not have as strong a relationship with Down syndrome as duodenal atresia**

The investigations confirm that baby Taylor has a ventricular septal defect (VSD).

Q **8. Describe the type of murmur that will be heard in a VSD in terms of where in the cardiac cycle it occurs. 1 mark**

A Pan- (½ mark) systolic (½ mark).

Q 9. What is an 'innocent murmur'? *1 mark*

A A functional murmur (½ mark), not associated with cardiac disease (½ mark).

📁 **LEARNING POINT**

Innocent murmurs
- **Soft, localised, systolic murmurs, not associated with a thrill**
- **Variation with posture and output status (heard in high-output states, ie children, pregnancy)**
- **Normal chest X-ray and echocardiogram**

The parents come to the paediatric cardiac clinic, with Baby Taylor, to discuss the diagnosis. Mr Taylor has been reading the patient information leaflet and also researching congenital heart disease on the Internet. He tells the consultant that he has been reading about 'blue babies' and asks if Baby Taylor will go blue.

Q 10. Name one cyanotic heart condition. *1 mark*

A 1 mark for any of the following:
- Tetralogy of Fallot^c
- Transposition of the great arteries
- Tricuspid atresia
- Total anomalous pulmonary venous drainage (TAVPD)

Q 11. Label this diagram of the fetal circulation. *4 marks*

A ½ mark each

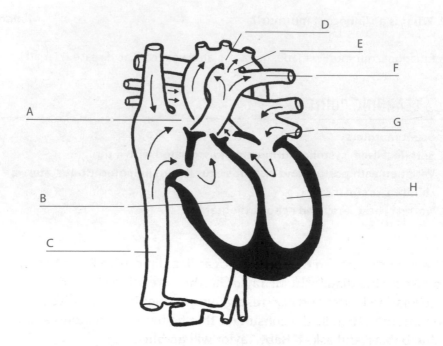

Figure 1.3: Fetal circulation.

A – Foramen ovale

B – Right ventricle

C – Inferior vena cava

D – Aorta

E – Ductus arteriosus

F – Pulmonary artery

G – Pulmonary vein

H – Left ventricle

Q **12. Explain the purpose of the ductus arteriosus.** *2 marks*

A The ductus arteriosus shunts blood from the pulmonary trunk to the arch of the aorta (1 mark) largely bypassing the fetal lungs (1 mark).

LEARNING POINT

The arrangement of the fetal circulation
- The fetal circulation is arranged to ensure maximally oxygenated blood reaches the fetal brain
- The blood entering the fetus from the umbilical vein is shunted past the liver in the ductus venosus and enters the inferior vena cava
- From the inferior vena cava the blood is projected through the right atrium in a direction which ensures it passes though the foramen ovale and thus into the left side of the heart, from where it is pumped to the fetal brain

Q 13. Describe the physiological changes to the circulation which occur at birth. *5 marks*

A All five bullet points must be represented in the answer for full marks:

- In the fetus, the left atrial pressure is low as relatively little blood returns from the lungs (½ mark). The pressure in the right atrium is higher than in the left, as it receives all the systemic venous return including blood from the placenta (½ mark).

- With the first breaths and expansion of the lungs (½ mark), resistance to pulmonary blood flow decreases (½ mark) and the volume of blood flowing through the lungs increases (½ mark).

- The increased pulmonary venous return leads to a rise in the left atrial pressure (½ mark). Meanwhile, the volume of blood returning to the right atrium falls (½ mark) as the placenta is excluded from the circulation (½ mark), decreasing the pressure in the right atrium (½ mark).

- The foramen ovale allows blood flow from the right to the left atrium in fetal life (½ mark). The change in the atrial pressures at birth causes the flap valve of the foramen ovale to close (½ mark).

- This results in the cessation of the large right-to-left shunt (½ mark), with consequent changes in blood gas levels (½ mark). Altered blood gas levels lead to smooth muscle contraction (½ mark) bringing about closure (½ mark) of the ductus arteriosus (½ mark), which connects the pulmonary artery to the aorta (½ mark) in fetal life. (This usually happens within hours or days.)

The consultant explains to Mr Taylor that a ventricular septal defect is not a 'blue baby' heart defect. It is one of the non-cyanotic heart conditions.

Q 14. The following are diagrams of non-cyanotic heart conditions. Please name each condition. *4 marks*

A

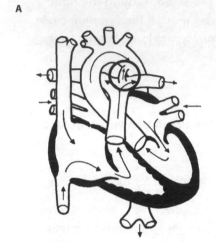

B

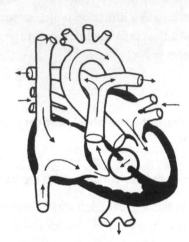

C

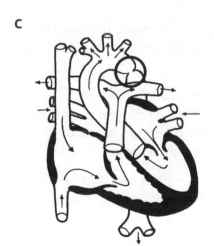

D

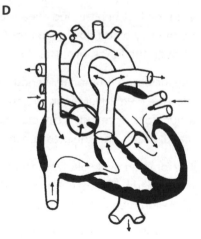

A – Patent ductus arteriosus

B – Ventricular septal defect

C – Coarctation of the aorta

D – Atrial septal defect or patent foramen ovale

The consultant explains that if the VSD is not repaired, it could develop into a cyanotic or 'blue' syndrome in later life, a phenomenon known as Eisenmenger's[d] syndrome. He tells the Taylors that unfortunately in the past children with Down syndrome often did not have their VSD repaired.

Q 15. Explain pathogenesis of Eisenmenger's syndrome (Why does the child go blue?)   *3 marks*

A All three bullet points must be represented in the answer for full marks:

- Conditions which can lead to Eisenmenger's syndrome are those associated with a left-to-right shunting of blood in the cardiac circulation (½ mark). The left-to-right shunt allows an increased volume of blood into the pulmonary circulation (½ mark), causing pulmonary hypertension (½ mark).

- Pulmonary hypertension damages the pulmonary artery wall (½ mark), which leads to further increases in pressure (½ mark) (or pulmonary vascular disease (PVD) (½ mark)). Eventually the pressure in the pulmonary arteries, and therefore the right ventricle, may increase such that it exceeds the pressure in the left ventricle (½ mark).

- When this occurs the shunt is reversed (½ mark) and de-oxygenated blood from the right side of the circulation is shunted towards the left (½ mark), resulting in a cyanotic condition (½ mark).

Mr and Mrs Taylor decide to go ahead with the surgery.

CARDIOLOGY

 BIBLIOGRAPHY

Forrester C, Carachi R, Goel K N, Young D G. 1996. *Children's Medicine and Surgery*. London: Arnold.

Haddad D F, Greene S A, Olver R E. 2000. *Core Paediatrics and Child Health*. Edinburgh: Churchill Livingstone.

Lissauer T, Clayden G. 2001. *Illustrated textbook of Paediatrics*, 2nd edn. London: Mosby.

 WEBSITES

American Heart Association: www.americanheart.org

Down syndrome UK: www.downs-syndrome.org.uk

Women's Health Information www.womens-health.co.uk/downs.asp

[a]John Langdon Down (1828–1896), English physician noted for his work with mentally retarded children. He described the features of Down Syndrome in 1866.

[b]Christian Doppler (1803–1853), Austrian mathematician and physicist, who described the Doppler effect, the apparent change in frequency and wavelength of a wave as perceived by an observer moving relative to the source of the wave.

[c]Etienne Fallot (1850–1911), French physician after whom Fallot's tetralogy is named. The condition had been described by Niels Stensen in 1672. Fallot was Professor of Hygiene and Legal Medicine in Marseille.

[d]Victor Eisenmenger (1864–1932), Austrian physician who described Eisenmenger's syndrome in 1897. The term was coined by Dr Paul Wood in 1958..

CARDIOLOGY
3. VALVULAR HEART DISEASE AND EMBOLISM

You are the Foundation Year 2 House Officer and are receiving for the medical team. Mr Smith, a 69-year-old man, has been referred by his GP with a suspected ischaemic right foot. The foot pain came on earlier in the day. Mr Smith has been complaining of fatigue, general malaise and breathlessness over the past few weeks, which has been gradually increasing and is worse on exertion. He had a myocardial infarction 2 years ago and made an uneventful recovery.

On examination you find that Mr Smith's right foot is pale and cool but there is no ulceration of the skin. You check the peripheral pulses. As you palpate each pulse you picture the artery running close to the bone.

Q 1. For each of the pulses given in the table below, select the bony site with which it is most closely associated from the following list. **3 marks**

Patella
Lower femur   Lateral malleolus

Upper tibia   Calcaneus

Head of fibula   Talus

Shaft of tibia   Navicular

Medial malleolus   Cuboid

Pulse	Associated region of bone
Popliteal	Lower femur (1 mark)
Posterior tibial	Medial malleolus (1 mark)
Dorsalis pedis	Navicular (1 mark)

The femoral pulse is present on the right side but no more distal pulses are palpable. All the pulses are palpable on the left side.

Q **2. Which is the most likely artery to have been obstructed?**   *1 mark*

A Femoral artery.

You carry out a general examination of the patient. You note that Mr Smith's radial pulse is 168 bpm and is irregularly irregular.

Q **3. What is this heart rhythm?**   *1 mark*

A Atrial fibrillation.

Q **4. Briefly outline the underlying electrical abnormality of the heart.**   *2 marks*

A Atrial fibrillation is characterised by chaotic atrial activity resulting in a lack of effective atrial contraction (1 mark). The atrial rate is so fast that many of the atrial impulses encounter refractory tissue at the atrioventricular (AV) node and cannot be conducted to the ventricles. Conduction of atrial impulses to the ventricles thus occurs irregularly (1 mark).

Q **5. In patients with an irregularly regular pulse, the pulse measured by auscultation of the apex beat is often faster than that measured at the radial pulse. What is this phenomenon called and explain why it happens?**   *2 marks*

A Pulse deficit (½ mark) – as the ventricular rate increases, diastolic filling time is reduced (½ mark). In atrial fibrillation, which is fast and irregular, the impulses can occur very close together. This means that there may be insufficient diastolic filling to create a cardiac output (no palpable pulse for that beat) (½ mark), but there has been enough blood flow to move the heart valves, so heart sounds are heard at the apex on auscultation (½ mark).

You now carry out a full examination of Mr Smith's cardiovascular system. On auscultation of the heart you hear a murmur. At this point you pause to review the cardiac cycle in order to help with your diagnosis.

Q 6. Here is a list of options of possible timings of events in the cardiac cycle relative to ventricular systole and diastole.

Option 1: Throughout ventricular systole

Option 2: Throughout ventricular diastole

Option 3: Early ventricular systole

Option 4: End of ventricular systole

Option 5: Early ventricular diastole

Option 6: End of ventricular diastole

Q In the table below give the timing option that best fits each event. The options may be used once, more than once, or not at all.　　*5 marks*

Event	Option
Flow into the ascending aorta	1
Opening of aortic valve	3
Closure of mitral valve	3
Closure of tricuspid valve	3
Flow through mitral valve	2

A 1 mark for each correct match

You listen again to Mr Smith's heart and confirm that you have heard a systolic murmur. It is best heard at the apex and radiates towards the axilla.

CARDIOLOGY

Q **7. What is the definition of a murmur?** *1 mark*

A A murmur is a sound generated by turbulent blood flow.

Q **8. The causes of systolic murmurs can be divided depending on whether they are ejection, pansystolic or late systolic. Insert the following causes of a systolic murmur into the appropriate lines in the table below. Each line in the answer box represents a different condition** *3 marks.*

Aortic stenosis

Mitral regurgitation

Mitral valve prolapse

Pulmonary stenosis

Tricuspid regurgitation

Ventricular septal defect

Ejection	Aortic stenosis
	Pulmonary stenosis
Pansystolic	Mitral regurgitation
	Tricuspid regurgitation
	Ventricular septal defect
Late systolic	Mitral valve prolapse

½ mark for each correct cause

Q 9. Identify A–J on the following diagram (Figure 1.4).   *5 marks*

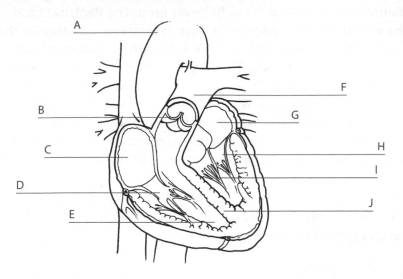

Figure 1.4: Anatomy of the heart

    A – Aorta

    B – Pulmonary valve

    C – Right atrium

    D – Tricuspid valve

    E – Right ventricle

    F – Pulmonary trunk

    G – Left atrium

    H – Mitral valve

    I – Chordae tendinae

    J – Interventricular septum

A ½ mark for each correct label.

You suspect that an embolus has formed due to the atrial fibrillation and passed to the right lower limb. The Registrar sends for the on-call vascular surgeon. A Doppler ultrasound confirms the diagnosis. The surgeon, plans to take Mr Smith to theatre to carry out an urgent embolectomy. The surgeon takes particular note of the time since the onset of the patient's foot symptoms. Had the ischaemia been prolonged he would have carried out fasciotomy, incision of the deep fascia bounding the osteofascial compartments of the lower limb. This is done to prevent muscular damage due to pressure caused by swelling of the contents of the compartments.

The diagram below (Figure 1.5) shows a cross-section through the calf and the osteofascial compartments: anterior, peroneal, superficial posterior and deep posterior.

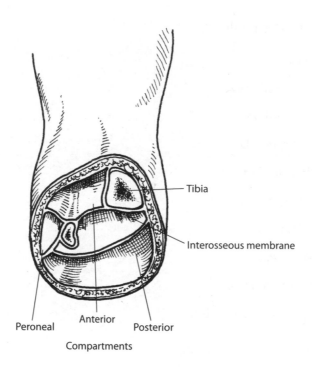

Figure 1.5: Cross-section through the calf and osteofascial compartments.

Q 10. In which compartment does each of the following muscles lie? *5½ marks*

Extensor digitorum longus

Extensor hallucis longus

Flexor hallucis longus

Flexor digitorum longus

Gastrocnemius

Peroneus brevis (fibularis brevis)

Peroneus longus (fibularis longus)

Peroneus tertius (fibularis tertius)

Soleus

Tibialis anterior

Tibialis posterior

Anterior compartment	Peroneal compartment	Superficial posterior compartment	Deep posterior compartment
Tibialis anterior	Peroneus longus	Gastrocnemius	Tibialis posterior
Extensor hallucis longus	Peroneus brevis	Soleus	Flexor digitorum longus
Extensor digitorum longus			Flexor hallucis longus
Peroneus tertius			

A ½ mark each

Q 11. Which nerve innervates the muscles in each of these compartments?

1½ marks

Anterior compartment	Peroneal compartment	Posterior compartment
Deep peroneal (fibular) nerve	Superficial peroneal (fibular) nerve	Tibial nerve

A ½ mark each

📖 BIBLIOGRAPHY

Levick J R. 2000. *An Introduction to Cardiovascular Physiology*, 3rd edn. London: Arnold Publishers

Longmore M, Wilkinson I, Torok E. 2001. *Oxford Handbook of Clinical Medicine*, 5th edn. Oxford: Oxford University Press.

CARDIOLOGY
4. MYOCARDIAL INFARCTION

You are the house officer on duty one evening in the Accident and Emergency Department when a 46-year-old man, Mr Clark, is brought in at 21.30 hours by the paramedic team from his home because of severe crushing central chest pain. He has no previous history of ill health. The pain started suddenly at around 19.30 hours while he was watching TV. You suspect that he has suffered a myocardial infarction.

Mr Clark complains of nausea and has vomited. He also tells you that his chest pain is radiating to his jaw and down his left arm. On examination, he is sweating and cold. He has a tachycardia and is breathless.

The autonomic nervous system is likely to be responsible for some of the symptoms and signs.

Q 1. Which division of the autonomic nervous system is likely to be responsible for the tachycardia, sweating and the cold peripheries? *1 mark*

A Sympathetic nervous system.

Q 2. Which cranial nerves are likely to be responsible for the nausea and vomiting? *1 mark*

A Vagus nerves.

Q 3. Which spinal nerves have their dermatomes: (a) in the anterior part of the neck and (b) in the upper limb? *2 marks*

a. Anterior neck: C2 (½ mark) – C4 (½ mark).

b. Upper limb: C5 (½ mark) – T2 (½ mark).

Q 4. Why does pain of cardiac origin radiate to the neck and to the upper limb? *4 marks*

A Nerve fibres that mediate the sense of pain from visceral structures generally run in cardiac nerves and with sympathetic fibres (1 mark). The neurons mediating pain from the heart thus enter the spinal cord through cervical (1 mark) and upper thoracic (1 mark) spinal nerves. The sense of pain is referred (1 mark) to regions of skin supplied by these spinal nerves.

Mr Clark has a 12 lead ECG carried out on arrival in the A & E Department.

A copy is shown in Figure 1.6.

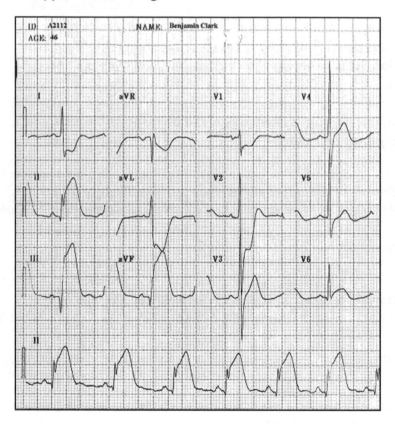

Figure 1.6: A 12-lead ECG.

Q 5. Calculate the heart rate. *1 mark*

A Heart rate is 70–85 beats /min.

 LEARNING POINT

Each large square represents 0.20 seconds and each small square 0.04 seconds. To calculate the heart rate as beats per *minute*, if the heart beat is regular, divide 1500 (ie 25×60) by the number of small squares between two consecutive equivalent waves. If irregular, measure several and give range.

Q 6. Mr Clark's ECG shows sinus rhythm. How can you tell? *2 marks*

A Regularly timed waveforms (1 mark), each starting with a P wave (1 mark).

 LEARNING POINT

Take a plain sheet of paper. Line it up against the trace and mark off each peak of a QRS complex. Move the piece of paper to another strip of same ECG; if rhythm is regular the marks will still fit the peaks on the paper.

Q 7. What is the pacemaker of the heart and where is it situated? *1 mark*

A The pacemaker of the heart is the sinoatrial node (½ mark). It lies in the myocardium on the right side of the right atrium close to its attachment to the superior vena cava (½ mark).

Q 8. If the pacemaker were isolated, its cells would discharge at the rate of about 100 per minute. Why is the resting heart rate slower than this? *1 mark*

A In the body, the vagal tone reduces the natural rate of the sinoatrial node to about 70 discharges per minute.

Q **9. In an ECG, what parts of the cardiac cycle are represented by the following:**

Q **9(a). The P-wave?**

Q **9(b). The P-Q interval?**

Q **9(c). The QRS complex**? *3 marks*

A a. The P-wave represents atrial depolarisation (1 mark).

A b. The P-Q interval represents the nodal delay in the atrioventricular node (1 mark).

A c. The QRS complex represents ventricular depolarisation (1 mark).

Q **10. What specific abnormalities are seen in the above ECG traces?** *2 marks*

- ST elevation in II, III, aVF and V6 (1 mark).
- ST depression in I, aVL, V1, V2 (1 mark).

Q **11. What is the diagnosis?** *3 marks*

A Acute (1 mark) inferior (1 mark) myocardial infarction (1 mark).

📁 **LEARNING POINT**

ST elevation in leads II, III and aVF indicates an inferior acute infarction.

Q **12. Identify by name each of the labelled blood vessels A–H on the diagram of the anterior view of the heart (Figure 1.7).** *4 marks*

A – Aorta (½ mark).

B – Left coronary artery (½ mark).

C – Pulmonary trunk/valve (½ mark).

D – Anterior interventricular branch of left coronary artery (left anterior descending coronary artery) (½ mark).

E – Posterior interventricular branch of right coronary artery (posterior descending coronary artery) (½ mark).

F – Circumflex branch of left coronary artery (½ mark).

G – Right coronary artery (½ mark).

H – Superior vena cava (½ mark).

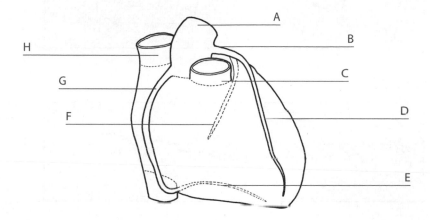

Figure 1.7: Anterior view of the heart.

Q **13. Identify on the diagram (with an X) the most likely site of arterial obstruction in this patient.** *1 mark*

A Anywhere on the right main coronary artery.

Shortly after the first ECG, at approximately 21.50 hours, Mr Clark suddenly vomited, had what the nurse described as a 'seizure' and became unconscious with no palpable pulses.

Lead II of his ECG was recorded at this point (Strip A).

This was followed shortly by the onset of a different rhythm (Strip B).

Q 14. Name the rhythm shown in each ECG (Figure 1.8). What was the heart rate in strip A? *3 marks*

Strip A

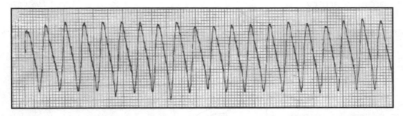

Strip B

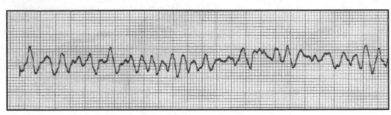

Figure 1.8: ECG.

A Rhythm in Strip A: ventricular tachycardia (1 mark): c. 250 discharges per minute (1 mark).

📂 LEARNING POINT

In rhythm A, the P-waves have been masked by the ventricular electrical activity.

A Rhythm in Strip B: ventricular fibrillation (1 mark).

Q 15. What would be the principal means used to resuscitate Mr Clark at this point? *1 mark*

A Defibrillation (½ mark) by DC (½ mark) electrical cardiac stimulation.

BIBLIOGRAPHY

Hampton J R. 2003. *The ECG Made Easy*, 6th edn. Edinburgh: Churchill Livingstone.

Kumar P, Clark M. 2005. *Clinical Medicine*, 6th edn. Edinburgh: Elsevier Saunders.

Williams P L. 1995. *Gray's Anatomy*, 38th edn. Edinburgh: Churchill Livingstone.

CARDIOLOGY
5. HEART FAILURE

You are the junior doctor on medical receiving on a busy Saturday night when you are called to the Accident and Emergency Department to see Mr Mayor, a 65-year-old retired teacher. Mr Mayor is gasping for breath, anxious and sweating. He is coughing up pink frothy sputum and on auscultation you hear crackling sounds, best heard as he breathes in. He is apyrexial. You diagnose acute pulmonary oedema and ask the nurses to ensure that he is kept sitting upright.

Q 1. List three treatments that you should give Mr Mayor at this stage. Include doses of any drugs. *3 marks*

A Any six of the following:

a. Oxygen (100% if there is no pre-existing lung disease) (½ mark).

b. Diamorphine IV (½ mark) 1– 2 mg slowly (½ mark) with an antiemetic (½ mark).

c. Furosemide IV slowly (½ mark) 20 mg (½ mark).

d. Consider IV glyceryl trinitrate infusion (½ mark), repeat dose of furosemide or IV aminophylline (½ mark) if refractory to initial treatment.

📂 LEARNING POINT

Acute pulmonary oedema is a medical emergency. It is essential to begin treatment before investigations. It is hard to distinguish between asthma, chronic obstructive pulmonary disease (COPD), pneumonia and pulmonary oedema clinically, especially in the elderly. If clinical diagnosis is uncertain, it is better to treat all the above simultaneously (eg with salbutamol, furosemide, diamorphine and amoxicillin).

Following your treatment, Mr Mayor is less breathless and you are able to take a more detailed history, carry out a thorough examination of the cardiovascular system and order necessary investigations. He tells you that he has had heart failure for the past 3 years following two myocardial infarctions in the past. He has smoked 20 cigarettes a day since he started teaching in his twenties.

You examine him carefully.

Q 2. List three symptoms and three signs of right and left heart failure in the table below. *6 marks; ½ mark each*

	Right heart failure	Left heart failure
Symptoms	Any three of the following (½ mark each): • Tiredness • Anorexia • Nausea • Bloated feeling	Any three of the following (½ mark each): • Dyspnoea • Orthopnoea • Paroxysmal nocturnal dyspnoea • Poor exercise tolerance • Fatigue • Wheeze • Nocturnal cough
Signs	Any three of the following (½ mark each): • Raised jugular venous pressure • Dependent pitting oedema • Cardiac cachexia • Tender smooth hepatomegaly • Ascites • Functional tricuspid regurgitation • Right ventricular heave	Any three of the following (½ mark each): • Pink-frothy sputum • Tachycardia • Displaced apex beat • Gallop rhythm • Fine crackles at lung bases • Functional mitral regurgitation

While you are arranging further investigations for Mr Mayor, the nurse hands you Mr Mayor's chest X-ray taken on admission.

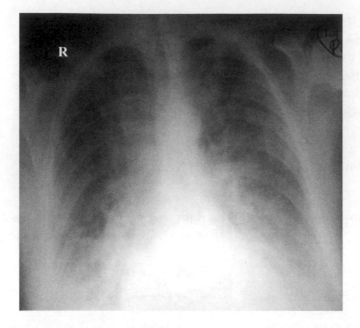

Figure 1.9: Mr Mayor's PA chest film.

Q **3. Give four characteristic features of heart failure that can be seen on this PA chest X-ray.** *4 marks*

A One mark each for any four of the following:

a. Cardiomegaly.

b. Kerley[a] B lines (interstitial oedema).

c. Enlarged hilum.

d. Upper lobe pulmonary diversion.

e. Bilateral pleural effusion.

f. Fluid in horizontal fissure.

You arrange for Mr Mayor to be admitted to the cardiology ward for specialist care. The next morning the medical student on a cardiology placement approaches you after the ward round and asks you to clarify some concepts regarding heart failure.

You remind her of the equation used to determine cardiac output:

Cardiac output = heart rate × stroke volume

Q 4. List three factors that could result in a fall in stroke volume, and hence in cardiac output. *1 mark*

A a. Preload reduced (¼ mark).

b. Myocardial contractility reduced (½ mark).

c. Afterload increased (¼ mark).

Q 5. The graph below illustrates the Frank[b]–Starling[c] Law.

Q 5(a). What is the Frank–Starling Law? *1 mark*

A The greater the end-diastolic volume, the greater the stroke volume.

Q 5(b). How does this relate to cardiac sarcomere configuration? *1 mark*

A Within normal limits, as the sarcomeres are stretched the functional contact between the myosin and actin filaments becomes more optimal thus increasing the force of contraction.

Use the graph (Figure 1.10) and the above equation to answer the following questions.

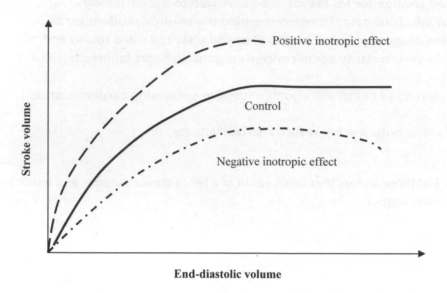

Figure 1.10: Relationship between end-diastolic volume and stroke volume.

Q **5(c). At a constant heart rate, what happens to cardiac output if venous return falls?** *1 mark*

A Cardiac output reduces.

Q **5(d). In cardiac failure, for a given heart rate and end-diastolic volume how does cardiac output compare to normal?** *1 mark*

A Cardiac output will be lower (negative inotropic effect through poor contractility).

Q **5(e). What happens to stroke volume if an increase in preload gives very high end-diastolic volumes?** *1 mark*

A No change (or possibly a fall) in stroke volume.

Q 5(f). In heart failure there is a downward shift of the ventricular performance curve. The reduced stroke volume results in incomplete chamber emptying during contraction. If in heart failure a weak ventricular systole gives incomplete chamber emptying, what will be the effect on the following ventricular systole? *1 mark*

A The next systole will be stronger.

Q 6. What is an inotrope and what is a chronotrope? *2 marks*

A An inotrope is an agent that alters the force of contraction of cardiac muscle (1 mark).

A A chronotrope is an agent that alters the heart rate (1 mark).

Q 7. Give an example of a positive inotrope and a positive chronotrope. *2 marks*

A Positive inotrope: calcium or digoxin or a catecholamine (1 mark).

A Positive chronotrope: a catecholamine or dopamine (1 mark).

Various pathophysiological changes occur in heart failure to compensate for the inability of the heart to pump sufficient blood to satisfy the needs of the body. Two of these are (a) salt and water retention and (b) stimulation of the sympathetic nervous system.

Salt and water retention is mediated by (a) the renin–angiotensin–aldosterone system and by (b) antidiuretic hormone.

Q 8. On which renal tubule cells do these two systems principally act? *2 marks*

	Tubules acted upon
Renin–angiotensin–aldosterone system	Principal cells of collecting ducts (1 mark)
Antidiuretic hormone	Collecting tubule/duct cells (1 mark)

Q 9. **Which receptors, by reduced stimulation, activate the sympathetic nervous system when there is a fall in systolic blood pressure?** *1 mark*

A The fall in blood pressure reduces discharge from baroreceptors in the carotid sinus (½ mark) and aortic arch (½ mark).

You reconsider the use of diuretics to address Mr Mayor's salt and water retention. You are familiar with bendroflumethiazide, furosemide and spironolactone.

Q 10. **In the following table indicate the class of diuretic to which each of these drugs belongs and indicate which acts at sites A, B and C on the diagram (Figure 1.11).** *3 marks*

	Class of diuretic
Bendroflumethiazide	Thiazide diuretic (½ mark)
Furosemide	Loop diuretic (½ mark)
Spironolactone	Potassium-sparing diuretic (½ mark)

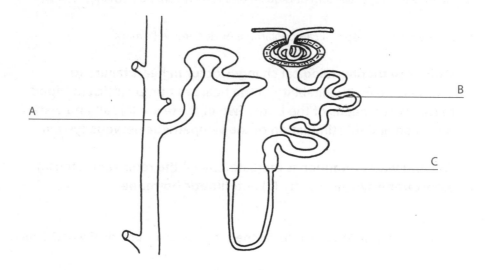

Figure 1.11: Site of drug action along the nephron.

A (½ mark for each)

A – Spironolactone.

B – Bendroflumethiazide.

C – Furosemide.

 LEARNING POINT

Amiloride is another example of a potassium-sparing diuretic and it blocks renal sodium uptake by acting on the distal convoluted tubules and collecting ducts.

You meet Mr Mayor in the canteen a couple of days later where he comes up to you to thank you. He mentions that he was very anxious during his admission and appreciated your support. You feel satisfied that you managed to diagnose and treat Mr Mayor effectively.

 BIBLIOGRAPHY

Guyton A C, Hall J E. 2006. *Textbook of Medical Physiology*, 11th edn. Philadelphia: Elsevier Saunders.

Kumar P, Clark M. 2005. *Clinical Medicine*, 6th edn. Edinburgh: Elsevier Saunders.

Longmore M, Wilkinson I, Turmeizi T, Cheung CK, Smith E. 2007. *Oxford Handbook of Clinical Medicine*, 7th edn. Oxford: Oxford University Press.

[a]Sir Peter Kerley (1900–1978), radiologist from Dundalk, Ireland, and a graduate of University College Dublin. He described several forms of line visible on chest X-rays in pathological conditions. He was Director of Radiology at the Westminster Hospital London.

[b]Otto Frank (1865–1944), German physiologist. He spent a short time in Glasgow but is particularly associated with the University of Munich and is remembered for his contribution to cardiac physiology.

[c]Ernest Starling (1866–1927), English physiologist, who worked at University College London. He is noted for the Frank–Starling Law, but he also discovered secretin and described the Starling Equation for fluid shifts.

CARDIOLOGY
6. VENOUS DRAINAGE OF THE LOWER LIMB

Miss McGuire, a 58-year-old woman, presents to you, her GP. Her complaint is varicose veins in both legs. She is having aching pains in both lower limbs but especially on her right side, the worse of the two. Her shop job entails being on her feet a lot and the ache is proving troublesome. She has tried wearing elasticated stockings and, while they helped for a while, the pain is becoming troublesome again.

Q 1. Where do the long (great) and short (small) saphenous veins lie in relation to (a) the ankle joint and (b) the knee joint. *4 marks*

A The long saphenous vein lies anterior to the medial malleolus at the ankle (1 mark) while the short saphenous vein lies posterior to the lateral malleolus (1 mark).

A The long saphenous vein lies posteromedial to the knee joint (1 mark). The short saphenous vein lies posterior to the knee joint (1 mark).

Q 2. In which veins do the two saphenous veins terminate? *2 marks*

A The long saphenous vein terminates in the femoral vein (1 mark). The short saphenous vein usually terminates in the popliteal vein (1 mark).

On examination of Miss McGuire's legs, the long saphenous vein on both sides and other nearby superficial veins are seen to be varicose. There is brown discoloration of the skin of the medial calf on the right limb. On the right leg, just above the medial malleolus and at the mid-point of the medial calf, the varicosities are particularly obvious and are forming raised nodules.

Q 3. What is the likely explanation for the two sites of marked varicosity? *1½ marks*

A These are likely to be sites of incompetent (½ mark) perforating veins (1 mark).

You also check for a saphena varix.

Q 4. Where is the 'saphenous opening'? *1 mark*

A In the upper (½ mark) medial thigh (½ mark).

Q 5. What is a saphena varix? *1 mark*

A A varicosity at the saphenous opening.

Q 6. Which muscle in the lower limb is particularly important in the return of venous blood from the lower limb and why is this? *3 marks*

A The soleus is an important postural muscle (1 mark). Within it are many veins that are squeezed (1 mark) as the muscle contracts (1 mark).

Q 7. Indicate which of the following groups of veins have valves. *1½ marks*

Veins	Yes or No
Superficial	Yes (½ mark)
Deep	Yes (½ mark)
Perforating	Yes (½ mark)

Q 8. What are venae comitantes? *2 marks*

A Paired veins (1 mark) that accompany arteries (1 mark).

In view of the pain and also the clinical appearance, you decide to refer Miss McGuire to the local hospital for surgical management of her varicose veins.

Later the same morning a second patient presents with venous problems in the lower limb. Mrs Campbell, a 54-year-old woman, comes in complaining of a 2-day history of acute onset of pain in her left calf. She is struggling to walk because of the pain. On further questioning you discover she returned from a shopping trip to New York one week ago. Examination reveals a tender, erythematous, swollen left calf and a normal right calf.

Mrs Campbell is referred to the local hospital for further investigation. A Doppler[a] ultrasound reveals a deep venous thrombosis (DVT).

Q 9. Using the terms below, fill in the boxes of the coagulation cascade (Figure 1.12). *4 marks*

Activated factor X

Activated factor XIII

Fibrinogen

Hard fibrin

Prothrombin

Prothrombinase

Soft fibrin

Thrombin

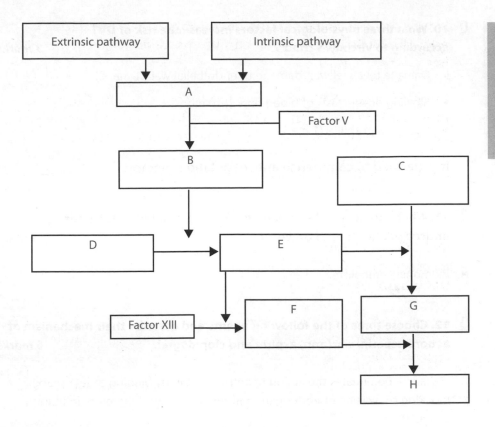

Figure 1.12: Coagulation cascade.

A ½ mark per box:

A – Activated factor X

B – Prothrombinase

C – Fibrinogen

D – Prothrombin

E – Thrombin

F – Activated factor XIII

G – Soft fibrin

H – Hard fibrin

Q 10. What three physiological factors increase the risk of DVT according to Virchow's triad[b]? *3 marks*

• Damage to vessel wall/damage to endothelial wall (1 mark).

• Slowing down/stasis of blood flow (1 mark).

• Hypercoagulability (1 mark).

It is decided to commence anticoagulation therapy.

Q 11. What potentially life-threatening complication of a DVT does anticoagulation aim to prevent? *1 mark*

A Pulmonary embolism.

Q 12. Choose three of the following agents and describe their mechanism of action: heparin, warfarin, aspirin and clopidogrel. *6 marks*

A Heparin – potentiates the action of anti-thrombin by binding to it (1 mark), blocking conversion of fibrinogen to fibrin (1 mark) and therefore inhibiting coagulation.

A Warfarin – prevents gamma carboxylation of vitamin K to its active form (vitamin K antagonist) (1 mark). Vitamin K is required in the synthesis of various clotting factors (II, VII, IX and X) in the liver (1 mark).

A Aspirin – an antiplatelet agent (1 mark). Prevents synthesis of thromboxane A_2 through inhibition of cyclooxygenase (COX) (1 mark). Thromboxane A_2 promotes platelet aggregation.

A Clopidogrel – inhibits ADP-receptor-mediated (1 mark) platelet aggregation (1 mark).

📖 BIBLIOGRAPHY

Ellis H. 2002. *Clinical Anatomy*, 10th edn. Oxford: Blackwell Publishing.

Kumar P, Clark M. 2005. *Clinical Medicine*, 6th edn. Edinburgh: Elsevier Saunders.

Sinnatamby C S. 1999. *Last's Anatomy: Regional and Applied*, 10th edn. Edinburgh: Churchill Livingstone.

[a]See Neurology Case 1.

[b]Rudolf Ludwig Karl Virchow (1821–1902), German doctor who made a number of medical discoveries including Virchow's node, an enlarged supraclavicular node indicative of upper gastrointestinal malignancy, and Virchow's triad, factors predisposing to deep venous thrombosis.

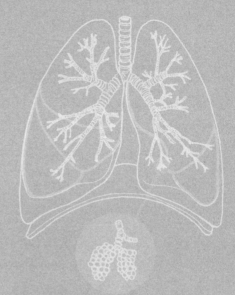

RESPIRATORY CASES: ANSWERS

RESPIRATORY
1. CYSTIC FIBROSIS

You are a final year medical student with the on-call house officer in Accident and Emergency and are asked to see a breathless young girl with a cough. You are surprised to learn that Lucy is 14 years old. She appears much smaller. Her mother tells you that she has cystic fibrosis. You feel alarm, but not panic, as you have yet to study this. You remember that consideration of basic science is important in understanding any clinical problem.

Cystic fibrosis affects a number of organs including the lungs. Lucy's mother says that she is worried Lucy has developed 'yet another chest infection' since starting a social support group with other children affected by cystic fibrosis.

🗁 LEARNING POINTS

Cystic fibrosis is a multi-system, progressive and variable disease.

Many fluid-secreting glands are affected, resulting in viscous secretions obstructing the pancreas, intestines and lungs. There is excess sodium chloride in the secretions from the sweat glands.

Pancreatic insufficiency leads to malabsorption of fat and fat-soluble vitamins. This results in steatorrhoea, poor weight gain and nutritional deficiency. Later this may be complicated by glucose intolerance and cystic-fibrosis-related diabetes mellitus.

Most males with cystic fibrosis are infertile. Inguinal hernia, hydrocele and undescended testes are more common. Females may also have reduced fertility.

Q 1. Label the diagram of the lungs below (Figure 2.1).   *6 marks*

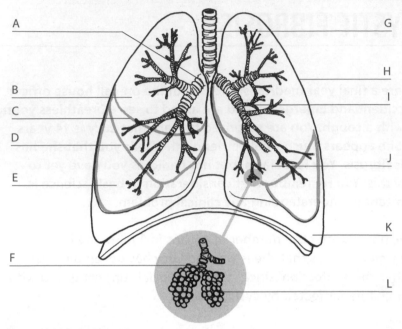

Figure 2.1: Anatomy of the lung.

A – Right main bronchus (½ mark).

B – Superior lobe –right lung (½ mark).

C – Horizontal fissure (½ mark).

D – Oblique fissure (½ mark).

E – Lower lobe – right lung (½ mark).

F – Respiratory bronchiole or alveolar duct (½ mark).

G – Trachea (½ mark).

H – Pleura (½ mark).

I – Left lower bronchus (½ mark).

J – Lingula (½ mark).

K – Costodiaphragmatic recess (½ mark).

L – Alveoli (½ mark).

You notice that Lucy is very breathless. As the house officer examines her chest you see muscles of her neck, chest and abdomen are moving as she struggles to take deep laboured breaths.

Q 2(a). **Name** *two* **accessory muscles of forced inspiration.** *2 marks*

A Any two of the following (1 mark for each):

- Pectoralis muscles

- External intercostals

- Scalene muscles

- Sternomastoid

Q 2(b). **Name** *four* **accessory muscles of forced expiration.** *2 marks*

A Any four of the following (½ mark for each):

- Rectus abdominis

- External oblique

- Internal oblique

- Transversus abdominis

- Internal intercostals

- Latissimus dorsi

- Abdominal muscles (½ mark if individual abdominal muscles above not given)

As you watch, Lucy gives a cough. As this happens, the lateral edge of a muscle becomes prominent on each side of her chest. The muscle edge is seen to run from the lower back to the humerus and to squeeze the chest as Lucy coughs.

Q 3. **Which muscle is this and what is its nerve supply?** *1 mark*

A Latissimus dorsi (½ mark).

Thoracodorsal nerve (½ mark).

Lucy has been coughing up copious sputum and a sample is collected for microbiological analysis. The house officer tells you that normal respiratory epithelial secretions contain a large number of chemo-protective agents such as lactoferrin and defensins. These help to prevent respiratory infections in healthy individuals.

Q 4. **Name** *two* **normal respiratory epithelial chemo-protective secretions (in addition to the two examples above).** *1 mark*

A Any two of the following (½ mark each):

- IgA

- Lysozyme

- Antiproteinase

- Antioxidants

- Surfactant proteins, eg collectins

- Secretory lactoperoxidase A2

- Lactoperoxidase

Q 5. **Name** *two* **cells of the innate immune system that you might expect to be present in Lucy's lung at this time.** *2 marks*

A Any two of the following (1 mark each):

- Macrophages

- Neutrophils

- Eosinophils

- Natural killer cells

- Mast cells

Infection seems likely and the house officer orders a chest x-ray. You anticipate being required to interpret the plain film and consider the relevant anatomy.

Here is the radiograph. It shows changes in the right upper lobe and consolidation in the middle part of the left lung field.

Q **6. Some normal anatomical features have been labelled. Please identify A–H.** *4 marks*

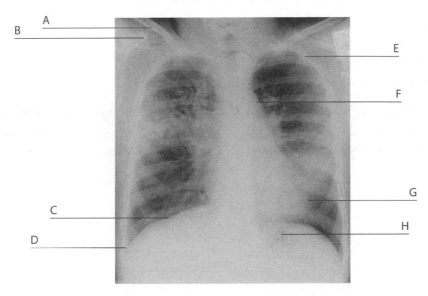

Figure 2.2: Lucy's chest radiograph.

A ½ mark for each of the following:

A – Clavicle.

B – Coracoid process.

C – Right dome of diaphragm.

D – Costophrenic angle.

E – Second rib.

F – Aortic knuckle (arch).

G – Left ventricle.

H – Fundus of stomach.

Meanwhile, Lucy's brother, 2-year-old Tom, is running riot around the Accident and Emergency Department. You wonder if he is also affected by cystic fibrosis. The doctor takes a family history and asks you to sketch a family tree into Lucy's case notes.

Q **7. Using the family history notes below, draw a family tree indicating:**

a. Lucy has cystic fibrosis.

b. Tom does not appear to have cystic fibrosis. (His 'Guthrie test' was negative. He has yet to have DNA analysis testing for cystic fibrosis genes.)

c. Their parents are both in good health.

d. Lucy's mother is expecting a third child, genotype unknown.

e. Lucy's maternal grandparents are both alive and well.

f. Lucy's uncle (mother's brother) died from cystic fibrosis, aged 24.   *4 marks*

A Award ½ mark for each correct note.

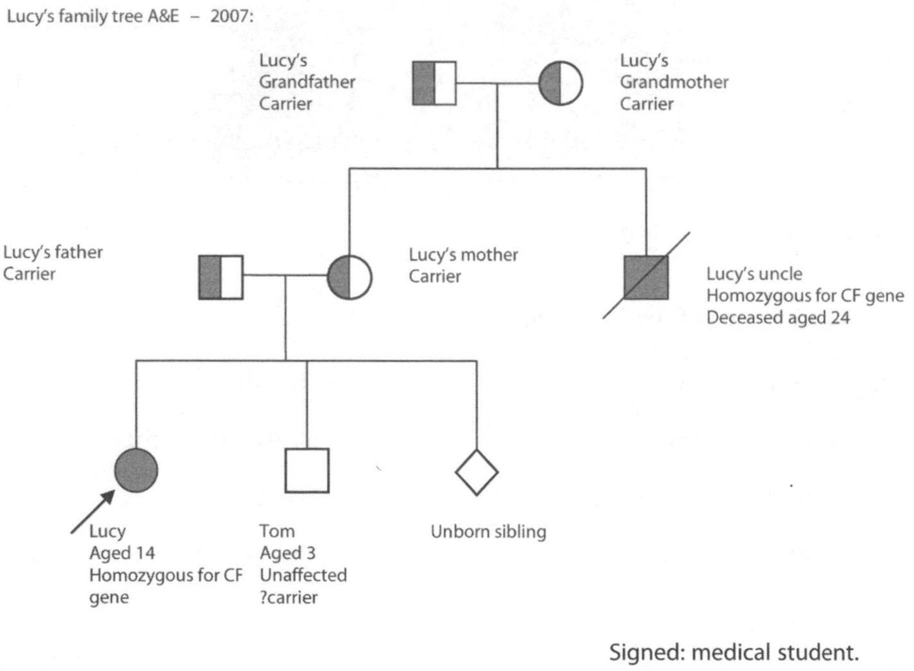

Lucy's family tree A&E – 2007:

Lucy's Grandfather Carrier

Lucy's Grandmother Carrier

Lucy's father Carrier

Lucy's mother Carrier

Lucy's uncle Homozygous for CF gene Deceased aged 24

Lucy Aged 14 Homozygous for CF gene

Tom Aged 3 Unaffected ?carrier

Unborn sibling

Signed: medical student.

Figure 2.3: Lucy's family tree.

Q **8. What is the Guthrie Test?** *2 marks*

A The Guthrie[a] Test was originally a screening test for phenylketonuria (1 mark). Blood collected by a pin prick (1 mark) shortly after birth is used to screen for phenylketonuria, but also for cystic fibrosis and hypothyroidism.

Q **9. State the mode of inheritance of cystic fibrosis.** *1 mark*

A Autosomal recessive.

Q **10. State the chance that Tom is a carrier for the gene mutation which causes cystic fibrosis.** *1 mark*

A One-half or 50%.

Q **11. State the chance that the unborn sibling will have cystic fibrosis.** *1 mark*

A One-quarter or 25%.

📁 LEARNING POINT

Cystic fibrosis is the UK's most common life-threatening inherited disease. Around 1 in 25 of UK Caucasians carries the gene mutation that causes cystic fibrosis.

Q **12. Define the term gene.** *1 mark*

A ½ mark each for any two of the following points:

- A gene is a sequence of DNA

- A collection of alleles

- Located on a specific chromosome

- Codes for a specific protein

RESPIRATORY

- May give rise to a specific phenotype

- Inherited from either parent

Q 13. What is the name of the protein affected by the gene defect, associated with cystic fibrosis? *1 mark*

- Cystic fibrosis transmembrane conductance regulator (1 mark)

- Allow CFTR (½ mark)

- Allow (cAMP-dependent) chloride channel (½ mark)

📁 LEARNING POINTS

Over 800 gene mutations have been identified in cystic fibrosis.

A gene located on chromosome 7 codes for the cystic fibrosis transmembrane conductance regulator (CFTR) protein.

In about 75% of cases the gene mutation named ΔF508 is found. This is a deletion of 3 DNA base pairs (1 codon) which results in phenylalanine being missing from amino acid position F508 in the final protein.

The CFTR is a cAMP-dependent chloride channel.

Q 14. Name the two ions affected by the defective protein in cystic fibrosis. *1 mark*

A Chloride (½ mark).

A Sodium (½ mark).

📁 LEARNING POINT

The chloride channel is one of several apical ion channels. It is found in the luminal membrane of epithelial cells in the conducting airways and on sweat-secreting epithelium. It controls the quantity and solute content of airway-lining fluid.

In cystic fibrosis the chloride transport protein is inactivated, resulting in reduced chloride secretion, absent inhibition of adjacent epithelial sodium channels and therefore excessive sodium resorption.

The result is dehydration of the airway lining and failure of reabsorption of NaCl from sweat.

Figure 2.4: The normal chloride channel and in cystic fibrosis.

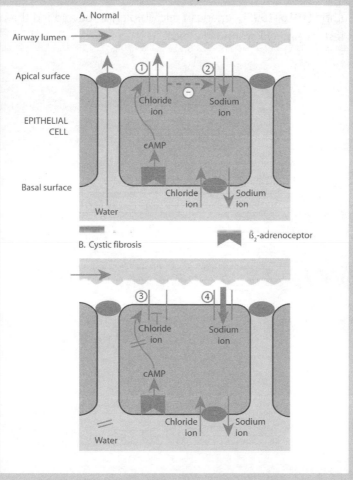

Lucy is admitted to the ward and started on intravenous antibiotics. You are pleased to see an improvement in her respiratory infection over the following few days.

RESPIRATORY

📖 BIBLIOGRAPHY

Boon N A, Colledge N R, Walker B R, Hunter J A A. 2006. *Davidson's Principles and Practices of Medicine*, 20th edn. Edinburgh: Elsevier Churchill Livingstone.

Hodson M, Geddes D, Bush A. 2007. *Cystic Fibrosis*, 3rd edn. London: Hodder Arnold.

[a]Robert Guthrie (1916–1995), American microbiologist, developed the neonatal screening test for phenylketonuria in 1961.

RESPIRATORY
2. TUBERCULOSIS

You are a locum GP in a busy practice in the middle of a morning surgery, when you are phoned by an anxious woman. Her father, 72-year-old Mr Stevens, has been quite unwell for over 2 weeks, and does not seem to be improving. He has a cough and a spit which is green at the moment and occasionally blood-stained. Recently, he has also been complaining of night sweats. Mr Stevens is reluctant to come and see you. He has a history of chronic obstructive pulmonary disease and suffers chest infections fairly regularly. He has told his daughter his chest has seemed worse in the past few months.

Q 1. Suggest four possible differential diagnoses.　　*2 marks*

A Any four of the following:

- Tuberculosis (½ mark)

- Infective exacerbation of COPD (½ mark)

- Pneumonia (½ mark)

- Bronchial carcinoma (½ mark)

- Pulmonary thromboembolism (½ mark)

After the discussion with his daughter you decide you should probably visit Mr Stevens. On your way over in the car you begin thinking about the anatomy and histology of the respiratory system.

Q **2. Identify A–C in this diagram of the end of a bronchiole (Figure 2.5).**

3 marks

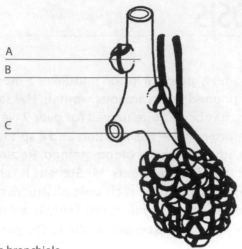

Figure 2.5: The bronchiole.

A 1 mark for each of:

A – Respiratory bronchiole

B – Pulmonary arteriole

C – Pulmonary venule

Q **3. Name the two main cell types found in the wall of an alveolus and describe their functions.** *2 marks*

A Type 1 pneumocytes – allow gaseous exchange/form blood–air barrier (1 mark).

A Type 2 pneumocytes – secrete surfactant (1 mark).

Q **4. At which stage of life are babies theoretically capable of respiratory survival because these cells begin functioning?** *1 mark*

A 28 weeks (surfactant develops).

You arrive at Mr Stevens's house to find him in bed, coughing, and very hot and clammy. He is coherent and you take a brief history from him. You discover he has been feeling like this for over 2 weeks, and has had frequent chest infections in the last year for which he has received antibiotics. He has a history of chronic obstructive pulmonary disease, hypertension and diabetes. He uses a fluticasone and salmeterol inhaler, and takes ramipril, aspirin and metformin. He has a vague memory of his grandfather having similar symptoms when he was a boy, but assumed it was because he was always smoking. Mr Stevens stopped smoking 5 years ago but smoked 30 cigarettes a day before that when he worked in the shipyard. He still enjoys a few whiskies.

Q 5. What is the rationale of the fluticasone and salmeterol in the inhaler? *2 marks*

A Fluticasone is a corticosteroid (½ mark) and has an anti-inflammatory action (½ mark).

A Salmeterol is a long-acting beta-2 adrenergic receptor agonist (½ mark) and thus is a bronchodilator (½ mark).

Q 6. Why is Mr Stevens taking ramipril and metformin and what types of drug are they? *2 marks*

A Mr Stevens is taking ramipril for hypertension (½ mark). It is an angiotensin-converting enzyme (ACE) inhibitor (½ mark). Metformin is a biguanide (½ mark) oral hypoglycaemic agent (½ mark).

On examination you find reduced bilateral air entry, reduced chest expansion, crackles in both bases and a small area of dullness over the right base.

Q 7. List four causes of a dull percussion note.   *2 marks*

A Any four of the following:

- Collapse   (½ mark)

- Consolidation   (½ mark)

- Effusion   (½ mark)

- Haemothorax   (½ mark)

- Chylothorax   (½ mark)

- Fibrosis   (½ mark)

You suspect Mr Stevens may have tuberculosis (TB) and he is admitted to hospital.

Q 8. Name the most likely causative organism.   *1 mark*

A *Mycobacterium tuberculosis.*

Q 9. Describe this organism   *4 marks*

Coccus or rod?	Rod (1 mark)
Aerobe or anaerobe?	Aerobe (1 mark)
Gram positive or Gram negative?	Gram positive (1 mark)
Produces spores/does not produce spores?	No spores (1 mark)

Q 10. What is the Ziehl-Neelsen stain?   *2 marks*

A Tubercle bacilli retain red (1 mark) coloration after histological specimens stained in carbol fuchsin are treated with acid alcohol, ie the bacilli are acid-fast (1 mark).

Mr Stevens is diagnosed as having pulmonary tuberculosis.

Q The consultant takes a group of students to see Mr Stevens. He asks them where they think he got tuberculosis. Since the patient is not aware of any TB contacts, they suggest secondary infection from someone that may not have been noticeably unwell, or reactivation due to his lowered immune status (COPD and diabetes). The consultant asks the students to think about primary TB infection in childhood.

Q 11. What name is given to the site of primary infection in the lungs? *1 mark*

A The 'Ghon[a] focus'.

Q 12. What is miliary tuberculosis? *1 mark*

A It is a disseminated form of tuberculosis that occurs if the bacilli enter and spread through the bloodstream.

Q 13. Name the type of immune response that occurs against tubercle bacilli. *1 mark*

A Delayed hypersensitivity *or* cell-mediated response *or* type IV hypersensitivity.

Q 14. What part of the organism triggers this reaction? *1 mark*

A Bacterial cell wall.

Below is a diagram of a chronic granuloma, typically associated with tuberculosis. It consists of a central necrotic core, surrounded by three cellular layers.

Q 15. The layers are labelled A–C. What is the general cellular content of each layer? *3 marks*

A 1 mark each for the following:

A – Macrophages

B – Lymphocytes

C – Fibroblasts

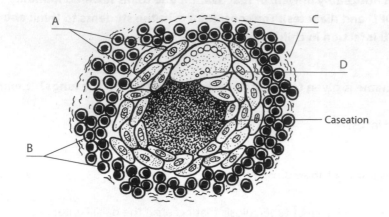

Figure 2.6: Chronic granuloma.

Q **16. A large cell is labelled D. What type is it?** *1 mark*

A Langhans[b] giant cell.

The students begin thinking about the fact that the body develops immunity to certain microbes and how science has used this to produce vaccines.

Q **17. Name the pre-vaccination test and the vaccination for tuberculosis.** *1 mark*

A Tuberculin skin test/Mantoux[c] test (½ mark).

A Bacille Calmette-Guerin[d] (BCG) vaccine (½ mark).

📖 BIBLIOGRAPHY

McMinn R M H, Gaddum-Rosse P, Hutchings R T, Logan B M. 1995. *Functional and Clinical Anatomy*. London: Mosby.

Reid R, Roberts F. 2005. *Pathology Illustrated*, 6th edn. Edinburgh: Churchill Livingstone.

Woolfe N, Wotherspoon A C, Young M. 2002. *Essentials of Pathology*. Edinburgh: W. B. Saunders.

[a]Anton Ghon (1866–1936), Austrian pathologist, who as a young man developed tuberculosis of the larynx but recovered. He is remembered for his work on tuberculosis and meningitis. Ghon eventually died from tuberculous pericarditis.

[b]Theodor Langhans (1839–1915), German pathologist and anatomist, described the multinucleated giant cell in 1867.

[c]Charles Mantoux (1877–1947), French physician, presented papers describing the Mantoux test (1908–1910).

[d]Albert Calmette (1863–1933), French physician, bacteriologist and immunologist. Worked at the Pasteur Institute. Studied attenuated *Mycobacteria* and snake venom. Camille Guerin (1872–1961) studied veterinary medicine and worked with Calmette in preparing antivenom against snake bites and vaccine against smallpox, as well as on attenuated *Mycobacteria* for protection against human and bovine tuberculosis.

RESPIRATORY
3. RESPIRATORY TRACT INFECTION

You are on duty in general practice one afternoon for urgent house calls when you are asked by the receptionist to visit 75-year-old Mr Gray, a widower living alone and normally very self-sufficient. His daughter, who lives about 50 miles away, has phoned the practice to say that she is very worried. Her father had had a bad cold and sore throat for a few days. Today he had sounded so strange on the telephone that she had driven over immediately. She had found her father to be confused, breathless, coughing and 'burning up'.

Q 1. Give the two most likely diagnoses to account for this presentation. *2 marks*

A Acute chest infection or acute pneumonia (1 mark).

A Delirium (1 mark).

You find Mr Gray, a thin man of moderate height, lying propped up in bed. He has a greyish, anxious appearance with a blue tinge to his lips and is difficult to rouse. Blood pressure is 110/70 mmHg, with a regular pulse rate of 108 beats per minute. His temperature is 40.5°C. Mr Gray has an increased respiratory rate and is using accessory muscles of respiration.

Q 2. What is the normal respiratory rate? *1 mark*

A The respiratory rate is normally about 10-20 breaths per minute (1 mark for value in this range).

Q 3. Which muscle is normally responsible for *quiet* inspiration? *1 mark*

A In quiet breathing the diaphragm is the principal inspiratory muscle.

 LEARNING POINT

The intercostal muscles stiffen the intercostal spaces and their role in moving the ribs becomes more important as breathing becomes more forceful.

Q 4. What mechanism brings about quiet expiration? *1 mark*

A Quiet expiration results from elastic recoil of the lung tissues.

Q 5. What are the main 'accessory muscles of respiration'? *2 marks*

A Sternocleidomastoid (1 mark).

A Pectoral muscles (1 mark).

Palpation revealed decreased expansion on the left side of the chest and increased vocal fremitus over the left base. Percussion revealed dullness over the left base.

Q 6. What is meant by the 'left lung base'? *1 mark*

A The lung base is the most inferior part of the lungs.

Q 7. Where does the lung base lie with respect to the surface anatomy of the chest wall? *1 mark*

A The lower limits of the lungs generally lie two ribs above the costal margin.

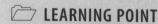

📁 LEARNING POINT

The costodiaphragmatic recess is the part of the pleural cavity that the lungs do not occupy and which extends to the costal margin between the diaphragmatic and costal pleurae. Posteriorly the lower limit of the recess lies between the 12th rib and the spinous process of T12.

Auscultation revealed bronchial breathing over the lower part of the left side of the chest along with generalised bilateral coarse crepitations and rhonchi. There was increased vocal resonance on the lower left side of the chest.

Q **8. What does increased vocal resonance indicate?** *1 mark*

A Increased vocal resonance at the left base indicates consolidation/collapse (1 mark) of the lung at the left base.

📁 LEARNING POINT

Air (tympanitic on percussion) is replaced by fluid/tissue (dull on percussion). Sound is conducted better through the fluid or tissue so the vocal resonance is increased.

Q **9. Identify A–F on the above radiograph (Figure 2.7).** *3 marks*

A – Coracoid process.

B – Right heart border/right atrium.

C – Right dome of diaphragm.

D – Costophrenic angle.

E – Clavicle.

F – First rib.

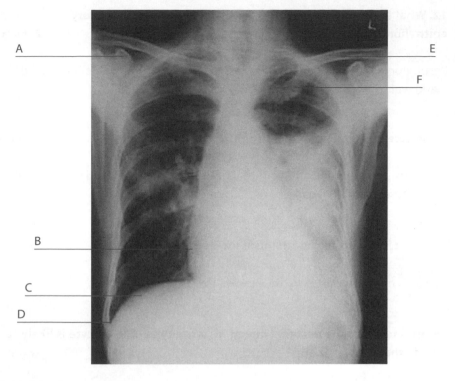

A

E

F

B

C

D

Figure 2.7: Chest radiograph.

Q **10. How can you tell that the patient's chest has been properly aligned to the x-ray plate?** *1 mark*

A The spinous processes of cervical vertebrae are visible in the midline of the tracheal shadow.

Q **11. Why, if possible, is a chest radiograph taken as a postero-anterior view, ie with the front of the patient's chest against the X-ray plate?** *1 mark*

A To minimise magnification of the image of the heart.

In this patient the diagnosis is pneumonia. It is usually precipitated by an upper respiratory tract infection, probably viral. This will have damaged the normal respiratory epithelium with loss of the mechanism for clearing mucus. Secondary bacterial infection is likely to have followed, with extension into the bronchioles and the alveolar spaces with the generation of an acute inflammatory reaction.

Q **12. What is the microscopical appearance of normal respiratory epithelium?** *2 marks*

A Respiratory epithelium is a pseudostratified (½ mark) columnar epithelium (½ mark) with ciliated cells (½ mark) and goblet cells (½ mark).

Q **13. Where does mucus in the respiratory tract come from?** *1 mark*

A The mucus comes from intra-epithelial goblet cells (½ mark) and from submucosal glands (½ mark).

Q **14. What is the normal mechanism for clearing the mucus?** *1 mark*

A Mucus is normally wafted up the airways towards the pharynx by cilia.

Q **15. As a result of the bacterial infection, what type of leukocyte is likely to invade the alveolar spaces?** *1 mark*

A Neutrophil polymorphs.

The host defences, which normally protect the lungs from infection, have obviously been overcome.

Q **16. List any four of these non-specific (innate) antimicrobial defence mechanisms in the respiratory tract.** *2 marks*

A Any four of the following (½ mark each):

- aerodynamic filtration
- cough reflex
- sneeze reflex
- mucociliary transport system
- phagocytic cells in alveoli (alveolar macrophages and polymorphs)
- complement

- cytokines

- natural killer cells

Because Mr Gray is living alone, is somewhat confused and has severe breathlessness and cyanosis, you arrange for him to be admitted to hospital. On admission arterial blood gases are checked on air. The results were as follows:

	[H⁺] (nmol/l)	$PaCO_2$ (kPa)	HCO_3 (mmol/l)	PaO_2 (kPa)	SaO_2 (%)
Reference range	36–44	4.6–6.0	22–28	10.5–13.5	>95
Mr Gray	61	4.0	11.8	6.8	79

Q 17. Explain these arterial blood gas findings on air. *3 marks*

A Any three of the following:

- Pneumonia leads to hypoxia because of ventilation–perfusion inequality in the area of lung with consolidation (1 mark). This area is perfused with blood, but no air (1 mark).

- Hypoxia results in metabolic acidosis (lactic acidosis), hence the H⁺ of 61 nmol/l (1 mark).

- Both acidosis and severe hypoxia (PaO_2 <8 kPa) stimulate the medullary respiratory centre via stimulation of peripheral chemoreceptors resulting in increased respiratory rate (1 mark) and hence a slight fall in $PaCO_2$ to 4.0 kPa (1 mark).

- Metabolic acidosis also uses up bicarbonate buffer in blood, so HCO_3 is reduced (1 mark).

Q 18. Where are the two main sites of peripheral chemoreceptors? *1 mark*

A The main peripheral chemoreceptors are the carotid bodies (½ mark), small structures that lie in the neck close to the bifurcation of the left and right common carotid artery and the aortic bodies (½ mark), which lie near the arch of the aorta.

Q 19. Which nerve(s) innervate these chemoreceptors? *1 mark*

A Carotid bodies are supplied by the glossopharyngeal nerve (½ mark); aortic bodies are supplied by the vagus nerve (½ mark).

Q 20. Describe the anatomical pathway of an oxygen molecule in a healthy lung as it diffuses from the alveolar gas to the haemoglobin molecule across the *thinnest* part of the blood air barrier. *2 marks*

A The oxygen molecule will cross the following layers at the thinnest part of the blood–air barrier:

- Type I pneumocyte (½ mark).

- Common basement membrane (½ mark).

- Capillary endothelium (½ mark).

- Red cell membrane (½ mark).

Q 21. Are lung capillaries fenestrated? *1 mark*

A No.

🗀 LEARNING POINT

Lung capillaries are non-fenestrated to prevent leakage of fluid into the alveoli.

📖 BIBLIOGRAPHY

Ganong W F. 2005. *Review of Medical Physiology*, 22nd edn. New York: McGraw-Hill Medical.

RESPIRATORY
4. ASTHMA

You are a house officer working in the acute receiving ward when Mr Roxburgh, a 35-year-old man, is admitted with sudden onset of severe left-sided chest pain and increasing shortness of breath. He is breathless with central cyanosis. Examination of the thorax shows decreased expansion on the left side which is hyper-resonant to percussion. The trachea is deviated to the right and the apex beat is palpable in the 5th intercostal space 1 cm from the left sternal edge.

His chest X-ray on admission is shown below

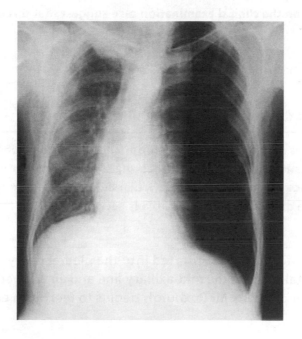

Q **1. What is the immediate cause of his acute symptoms?** *2 marks*

A Tension (1 mark) pneumothorax (1 mark).

His systolic blood pressure is 100 mmHg.

Q **2. What might this measurement indicate?**   *1 mark*

A Cardiogenic shock (1 mark).

A Shock alone (½ mark).

📂 **LEARNING POINT**

Cardiogenic shock occurs when, for whatever reason, tissue perfusion is impaired because the heart is not able to pump effectively. In this patient the tension pneumothorax is pressing on the heart and great vessels, impairing the pumping action.

Q **3. The radiograph shows that the mediastinum has shifted. What two findings on the clinical examination also suggest that this has occurred?**   *2 marks*

A The displaced trachea (1 mark) and apex beat (1 mark).

📂 **LEARNING POINT**

The apex beat is defined as the most inferior and lateral point where the apex beat is distinctly palpable. In the healthy adult it should be in the 5th intercostal space just within the midclavicular line. This is almost invariably on the left side of the chest; dextrocardia is very rare (<0.5%).

A wide-bore needle is now inserted into the pleural cavity via the 6th intercostal space in the mid-axillary line and air allowed to escape under pressure. Mr Roxburgh begins to feel much easier.

Q **4. What is the pleural cavity?**   *1 mark*

A The pleural cavity is the potential space (½ mark) between the visceral and parietal layers of the pleura (½ mark).

Q **5. What is the costodiaphragmatic recess?** *1 mark*

A The inferior recess of the pleural cavity, which is not occupied by the lungs (1 mark).

Or

A The recess between the costal and diaphragmatic pleurae (1 mark).

Q **6. In Mr Roxburgh, the pressure in the pleural cavity had risen. Which of the following is the most likely mean intrapleural pressure in a normal subject?** *1 mark*

A – –6 cmH$_2$O

B – 0 cmH$_2$O

C – 10 cmH$_2$O

D – 760 cmH$_2$O

A A – –6 cmH$_2$O.

As well as breathlessness, Mr Roxburgh complains of pleuritic-type chest pain.

Q **7. From which particular tissue layer is the pain arising?** *1 mark*

A Parietal pleura (1 mark).

A Pleura alone gets no marks.

After air had been allowed out of the pleural cavity, a water seal drain, inserted as before, replaced the needle.

Q **8. Name four muscles that the drain will penetrate.** *2 marks*

A ½ mark for each:

- Serratus anterior.

- External intercostal.

- Internal intercostal.

- Innermost intercostal.

Q 9. Other than the muscles, what structures are at risk in: (a) the upper part of the intercostal space and (b) the lower part of the intercostal space? *2 marks*

a. Upper part: the intercostal nerve (½ mark) and vessels (½ mark) or artery and vein (½ mark) in the uppermost part of the space.

b. Lower part: the collateral branches of the vessels (1 mark) in the lower part of the space.

You now discover that Mr Roxburgh is an asthmatic and had had an exacerbation of this the day before he became acutely breathless.

After he has recovered from his acute asthma and from his pneumothorax he has respiratory function tests carried out.

Q 10. On the following diagram of lung volumes (Figure 2.8), which functional parameters are represented by labels I, II and III? *3 marks*

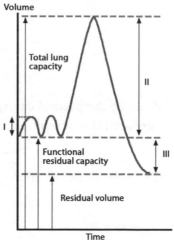

Figure 2.8: Lung volumes.

A 1 mark for each of the following:

I – Tidal volume

II – Inspiratory capacity

III – Expiratory reserve volume

Q **11. How is total lung capacity defined?** *1 mark*

A The total volume of the lung after maximum inspiration.

Q **12. Approximately what is the normal total lung capacity in a male adult?** *1 mark*

A About 6 litres.

A report comes back from the Pulmonary Function Laboratory with the values shown in the table below.

Lung volumes	Normal ref range	Patient	Patient after bronchodilator
FEV 1 (litres)	4.0	2.3	3.5
FVC (litres)	5.0	4.1	4.8
FEV/FVC	80%	56%	73%

Q **13. Define the terms FEV and FVC as used here.** *2 marks*

A FEV – Forced expiratory volume of gas exhaled in 1 second by a forced expiration from total lung capacity (1 mark).

A FVC – Total volume of gas that can be exhaled by forced expiration (1 mark).

Q **14. Explain the findings** *3 marks*

A The patient has objective evidence of moderate airways obstruction (1 mark), but this is largely reversible after inhaled bronchodilator (1 mark). These findings are consistent with the diagnosis of asthma (1 mark).

Q 15. To which of the following levels of the respiratory tract do smooth muscle fibres extend? *1 mark*

Portion of airway	Smooth muscle present?
Lobar bronchi	Yes
Segmental bronchi	Yes
Terminal bronchioles	Yes
Respiratory bronchioles	Yes
Alveolar walls	No

Q 16. How are the smooth muscle fibres orientated in the smaller airways? *1 mark*

A Spirals.

Q 17. In asthma, name two of the major cell types responsible for the release of chemical mediators that cause bronchial smooth muscle to contract. *1 mark*

A Mast cells (½ mark).

A Eosinophils (½ mark).

Mr Roxburgh has a history consistent with atopic asthma.

Q 18. What type of hypersensitivity response is this? *1 mark*

A Type I hypersensitivity.

Prior to this episode Mr Roxburgh used regular inhaled salbutamol to control his asthma symptoms.

Q 19. What is the mode of action of this drug? *1 mark*

A Salbutamol is a beta$_2$ adrenoreceptor (½ mark) agonist/stimulant (½ mark).

During this episode he required oral steroids as well and it is decided to discharge him on a combination treatment, 'Symbicort' – budesonide and formoterol fumarate.

Q 20. What is the mode of action of each of these? *2 marks*

A Budesonide – Steroid. Inhibits inflammatory/immune response (1 mark).

A Formoteral – Beta$_2$ receptor agonist promoting bronchodilatation (1 mark).

📖 BIBLIOGRAPHY

Ganong W F. 2005. *Review of Medical Physiology*, 22nd edn. New York: McGraw-Hill Medical.

Kumar P, Clark M. 2005. *Clinical Medicine*, 6th edn. Edinburgh: Elsevier Saunders.

West J B. 2001. *Pulmonary Physiology and Pathophysiology: An Integrated Case-Based Approach*. Philadelphia: Lippincott, Williams and Wilkins.

RESPIRATORY

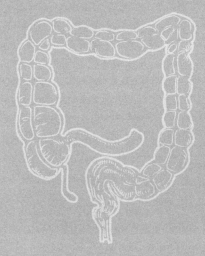

GASTROENTEROLOGY CASES:
ANSWERS

GASTROENTEROLOGY
1. EPIGASTRIC PAIN

Mrs Jones, a 43-year-old woman, has been admitted to the Accident and Emergency Department with sudden onset of severe pain in the epigastric region which radiated through to her back. She complains of feeling nauseous and has vomited twice. On examination, she is pale and her sclerae are jaundiced. She is tachycardic with a pulse rate of 110 beats per minute. Her blood pressure is 90/60 mmHg. Abdominal examination reveals ecchymosis of the flanks, tenderness in the epigastric area and bowel sounds are present. You suspect acute pancreatitis.

Q 1. Label this diagram of structures in the upper abdomen (Figure 3.1). *3 marks*

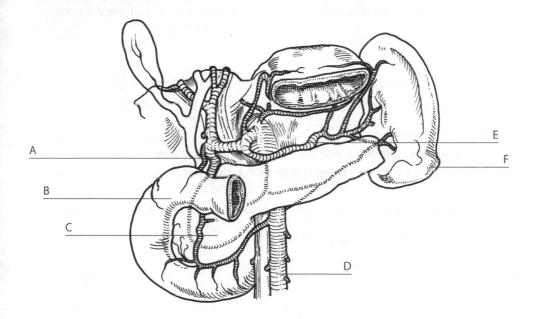

Figure 3.1: Anatomy of the upper abdomen.

A ½ mark per correct label (3 marks in total):

A – Gastroduodenal artery

B – Duodenum

C – Head of pancreas

D – Superior mesenteric artery

E – Splenic artery

F – Spleen

📂 **LEARNING POINT**

The pancreas is a retroperitoneal, hook-shaped organ about 15 cm long. The head of the pancreas lies within the C-shape of the duodenum, while the tail of the pancreas lies anterior to the hilum of the left kidney and extends to the hilum of the spleen. The main blood supply to the pancreas is via the splenic artery, a branch of the coeliac trunk. The splenic artery supplies the neck, body and tail of the pancreas. The head is supplied by the superior and inferior pancreatoduodenal arteries. Venous drainage is mainly via the splenic vein.

Blood tests reveal high serum amylase levels and raised blood glucose, supporting your suspicions of acute pancreatitis.

Q 2. Name four individual principal enzymes produced by the exocrine pancreas and state the foodstuff on which they act.   *4 marks*

A 1 mark for the name of the enzyme and the correct substrate (4 marks in total):

Enzyme	Substrate
Amylase	Starch
Lipase	Lipids
Trypsin	Protein
Chymotrypsin	Protein
Elastase	Protein

📂 LEARNING POINT

Trypsinogen and chymotrypsinogen are zymogens or proenzymes. Most of the proteolytic enzymes are stored this way to avoid self-digestion. They are secreted from the pancreas into the duodenum. Trypsinogen is cleaved by brush border enzymes into its active form, trypsin. Chymotrypsinogen is converted to chymotrypsin by trypsin.

Further investigation with an ultrasound reveals dilation of the biliary tree, which you suspect to be due to impaction of a gall stone in the common bile duct.

Q 3. Label this diagram of the biliary tree (Figure 3.2). *4 marks*

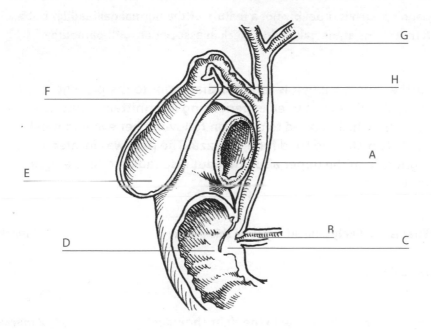

Figure 3.2: The biliary tree.

A ½ mark for each correct label, 4 marks in total:

A – Common bile duct

B – Pancreatic duct

C – Hepatopancreatic ampulla

D – Major duodenal papilla

E – Fundus of gallbladder

F – Cystic duct

G – Left hepatic duct

H – Hartmann's pouch

📂 LEARNING POINT

Hartmann's pouch is probably not a feature of the normal gallbladder but a pouch that forms at the gallbladder neck in association with pathology.

On further questioning it is revealed that, prior to the present episode, Mrs Jones has been experiencing intermittent bouts of colicky pain which tended to come on following her evening meal, particularly if she had fried food or pizza. The pain was located in the right side of the upper abdomen but also radiated to the right shoulder area.

Q 4. What is the likely clinical cause of this pain? *1 mark*

A Cholecystitis.

Q 5. Why does the pain radiate to the right shoulder? *2 marks*

A This is referred pain. The phrenic nerve (1 mark) gives sensory fibres to the adjacent diaphragm and possibly to the gallbladder. Many of the fibres come from C4 spinal nerve (1 mark) which is also sensory to the shoulder.

Q **6. Explain the hormonal control of gallbladder contraction.** *1 mark*

A Cholecystokinin (CCK) (½ mark) release is stimulated by the presence of fatty and acidic chyme (½ mark) in the small intestine, causing the gallbladder to contract.

Along with the amylase and glucose results the following results of liver function tests are received.

Blood results:

Test	Alkaline phosphatase	Alanine transaminase	Bilirubin	Conjugated bilirubin
Result	1832 U/l (39–117 U/l)	186 U/l (5–40 U/l)	204 µmol/l (< 17 µmol/l)	166 µmol/l

Q **7. The biochemistry results indicate that Mrs Jones has obstructive (post-hepatic) jaundice. Explain the reasoning that leads to this diagnosis.** *3 marks*

A Bilirubin is mainly conjugated in the liver. Most of the bilirubin is conjugated (1 mark) so it must have passed though the liver (1 mark). Alkaline phosphatase is produced by the epithelial lining of the bile ducts and raised levels indicate obstruction (1 mark).

▱ LEARNING POINT

Jaundice reflects a raised serum bilirubin concentration. It is usually clinically evident when greater than twice the normal level.

Q **8. Bilirubin is formed from haem during the destruction of old or damaged erythrocytes in the spleen. Please answer the following questions on bilirubin metabolism after it leaves the spleen. Each question is worth ½ mark.** *4 marks*

345

Q 8(a). Is the bilirubin produced by the spleen soluble in water?

A No (½ mark).

Q 8(b). To which substance is bilirubin bound as it is passed in the venous blood from the spleen to the liver?

A Albumin (½ mark).

Q 8(c). By which two veins does the bound bilirubin pass from the spleen to the liver?

A Splenic and portal veins (½ mark: must give both).

Q 8(d). Which cell organelle is responsible for conjugation of bilirubin?

A Endoplasmic reticulum (½ mark).

Q 8(e). Into which lumen is conjugated bilirubin directly secreted by hepatocytes?

A Bile canaliculus (½ mark).

Q 8(f). What is the source of the enzymes that reduce bilirubin to urobilinogen in the bowel?

A Bacteria (½ mark).

Q 8(g). Which vein carries resorbed urobilinogen from the terminal ileum to the portal vein?

A Superior mesenteric vein (½ mark).

Q 8(h). As well as loss in the stools, by what other means is urobilinogen lost from the body?

A In urine (½ mark).

Having presented with jaundice, Mrs Jones underwent urgent endoscopic retrograde cholangiopancreatography (ERCP). This confirmed the presence of a gallstone impacted in the common bile duct, which was subsequently removed. The stone was mainly composed of cholesterol.

Q 9. Give two functions of cholesterol?   *2 marks*

A Any two of the following (1 mark each):

- Precursor of steroid hormones, eg aldosterone, cortisol, progesterone, oestrogen and testosterone

- Component of cell membranes/repair of cell membranes

- Precursor of bile acids

- Component of plasma lipoproteins

During her admission Mrs Jones had a CT scan with contrast to exclude pancreatic necrosis or abscess formation. Below is a CT scan of a normal upper abdomen.

GASTROENTEROLOGY

Q 10. Identify structures A–H (Figure 3.3). *4 marks*

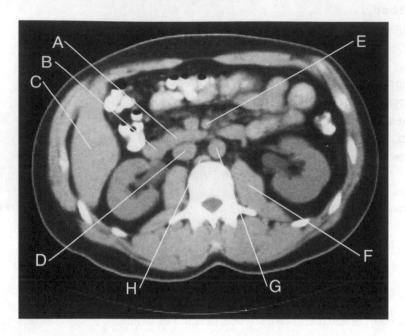

Figure 3.3: CT of abdomen.

A 4 marks total – ½ mark each:

A – Head of pancreas

B – Duodenum

C – Liver

D – Interior vena cava

E – Superior mesenteric artery

F – Psoas major muscle

G – Aorta

H – Right crus of diaphragm

Mrs Jones was managed conservatively with fluids, analgesia and her hyperglycaemia was corrected using insulin. Before discharge she is started on a statin.

Q 11. Explain how statins work.   *2 marks*

A Statins competitively inhibit the action of HMG-CoA reductase, reducing hepatic cholesterol synthesis (1 mark) but they also induce LDL-receptor expression and therefore enhance cholesterol clearance by the liver (1 mark).

📖 BIBLIOGRAPHY

Boon N A, Colledge N R, Walker B R, Hunter J A A. 2006. *Davidson's Principles and Practices of Medicine*, 20th edn. Edinburgh: Elsevier Churchill Livingstone.

Burkitt H G, Quick C R G. 2002. *Essential Surgery: Problems, Diagnosis and Management*. Edinburgh: Churchill Livingstone.

Garden O, Bradbury A, Forsythe J. 2002. *Principles and Practice of Surgery*, 4th edn. Edinburgh: Elsevier.

Kumar P, Clark M. 2005. *Clinical Medicine*, 6th edn. Edinburgh: Elsevier Saunders.

Pocock G, Richards C. 2004. Human Physiology: The Basis of Medicine, 2nd edn. Oxford Core Texts.

GASTROENTEROLOGY
2. INFLAMMATORY BOWEL DISEASE

Mr McDonald, a 29-year-old plumber, presents to his GP with a 2-week history of bloody diarrhoea and abdominal pain. He has been feeling generally unwell but has not experienced vomiting. On further questioning he tells his GP he has been passing stools 5–6 times per day and has also been passing mucus. Mr McDonald has not lost any weight recently but his appetite has been reduced. At this stage, two main differential diagnoses are considered, inflammatory bowel disease (IBD) and infection. There was no history of overseas travel.

On initial examination, there is mild peri-umbilical tenderness and blood and mucus are identified on rectal examination. A stool sample is collected and sent for microbiological analysis.

Q 1. **Name four organisms which commonly cause bloody diarrhoea.** *2 marks*

A ½ mark each for any four of the following:

- *Escherichia coli*

- *Shigella* species

- *Salmonella* species

- *Campylobacter* species

- *Entamoeba histolytica* (amoebic dysentery)

Stool sample results are negative and Mr McDonald continues to suffer from bloody diarrhoea. Routine blood tests are taken at initial presentation including full blood count, urea and electrolytes and C-reactive protein (CRP).

The results are as follows:

	Mr McDonald's results	Normal range
Hb	10.3 g/dl	12.5–16.5 g/dl
MCV	88 fl	83–101 fl
WCC	$12.2\times10^9\,l^{-1}$	$(4.0–11.0)\times10^9\,l^{-1}$
Platelets	$296\times10^9\,l^{-1}$	$(150–400)\times10^9\,l^{-1}$
CRP	64 mg/l	<10 mg/l

A blood film is also examined and the erythrocytes appear normal.

Q **2(a). Where is CRP produced?**   *1 mark*

A CRP is produced by the hepatocytes.

Q **2(b). What is the clinical significance of elevated CRP?**   *1 mark*

A When raised, it is a non-specific indicator of inflammation or infection in the body (1 mark), or it is an acute phase reactant protein (1 mark).

Q **3. What type of anaemia is this?**   *1 mark*

A Normochromic (½ mark), normocytic anaemia (½ mark).

Anaemia of chronic disease also accepted (1 mark).

Due to the presence of anaemia, tests of serum ferritin, folate, B_{12} and iron are requested. B_{12}, folate and iron are found to be low and ferritin levels are raised. When body iron stores are low, ferritin production is usually down-regulated.

Q **4(a). Why is the ferritin level elevated in this patient?**   *1 mark*

A Ferritin is also an acute phase reactant produced by the liver and is elevated in times of illness or inflammation (1 mark).

Q **4(b). What ionic form of iron is most commonly ingested, ferric or ferrous?** *1 mark*

A Most iron ingested is in the form of Fe^{3+} (ferric iron).

Q **4(c). What ionic form of iron is absorbed in the GI tract?** *1 mark*

A Fe^{2+} (ferrous iron).

 LEARNING POINT

Fe^{3+} is converted to Fe^{2+} by enzymes on the brush border of enterocytes.

Q **4(d). Where in the gastrointestinal tract does iron absorption occur?** *1 mark*

A Iron absorption occurs in the duodenum.

Q **4(e). How is iron transported into cells and what is its fate after this?** *4 marks*

A Fe^{2+} is transported into the enterocyte (½ mark) by DMT-1 (divalent metal transporter) (½ mark).

It can then either be stored in the enterocyte as ferritin if body iron stores are high (½ mark) or it can be transported out of the cell by ferroportin, a transporter in the basolateral membrane (½ mark).

In plasma, Fe^{2+} is converted back to Fe^{3+} (½ mark) and binds to transferrin (½ mark).

It is then carried to sites such as the liver (½ mark), bone marrow (½ mark) and spleen (½ mark).

A colonoscopy is arranged for Mr McDonald.

Q 5(a). List the four main histological layers of the colon.   *2 marks*

A Mucosa (½ mark)

Submucosa (½ mark)

Muscularis externa (½ mark)

Serosa/adventitia (½ mark)

Q 5(b). The longitudinal muscle fibres of the muscularis externa of the colon are arranged into three bands in the colon. What are these called?   *1 mark*

A Taeniae coli.

Q 5(c). Between which layers would you find the myenteric plexus (Auerbach's plexus)?   *1 mark*

A Circular and longitudinal muscle layers.

📁 LEARNING POINT

The intestine is innervated by the autonomic nervous system.

Parasympathetic cholinergic activity increases the activity of intestinal smooth muscle. **Sympathetic noradrenergic activity** decreases activity of intestinal smooth muscle and causes sphincters to contract.

There are two major networks of nerve fibres in the GI tract:
- Submucous plexus: found in submucosa, also known as Meissner's plexus.
- Myenteric plexus: found in muscularis between circular and longitudinal muscle layers, also known as Auerbach's plexus.

The parasympathetic supply to the intestine ends on postganglionic neurons of the submucous and myenteric plexuses.

Sympathetic fibres reaching the bowel are postganglionic neurons and end directly on smooth muscle cells.

Biopsies of the colon were taken and histology results are awaited.

Q 6(a). The colon is illustrated below (Figure 3.4). Identify
structures A to H.   *4 marks*

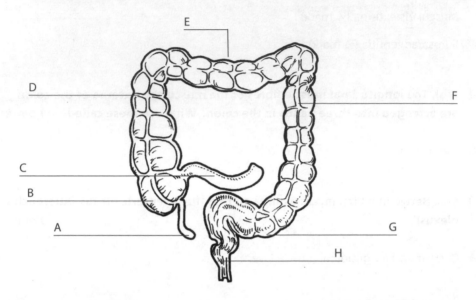

Figure 3.4: Diagram of colon.

A ½ mark for each of the following:

A – Appendix

B – Caecum

C – Terminal ileum

D – Ascending colon

E – Transverse colon

F – Descending colon

G – Sigmoid colon

H – Rectum

Q 6(b). List two of these structures that are retroperitoneal. *1 mark*

A Ascending colon, descending colon, rectum (½ mark for any two).

Q 6(c). Name one other retroperitoneal structure. *1 mark*

A Kidney, adrenal gland, duodenum, pancreas, ureter, inferior vena cava (IVC), aorta, oesophagus.

A Only part of the duodenum and oesophagus are retroperitoneal (either of these should receive ½ mark).

Q 6(d). What is the blood supply of the ascending colon? *1 mark*

A Superior mesenteric artery or ileocolic artery and right colic artery.

During colonoscopy, the macroscopic appearance is suggestive of inflammatory bowel disease (IBD) with diffuse bleeding and inflammation. The two main subgroups of IBD are ulcerative colitis and Crohn's disease.

Q 7. Complete the following table relating to pathological differences between ulcerative colitis and Crohn's disease. *5 marks*

	Crohn's disease	Ulcerative colitis
Part of GI tract affected	Any part of GI tract from mouth to anus (½ mark)	Colon and rectum only (½ mark)
Are the lesions continuous?	No – skip lesions (½ mark)	Yes – continuous through colon and rectum (½ mark)
Which layers of the gut wall are affected?	Transmural – all layers (½ mark)	Mucosa (½ mark)
How are goblet cell numbers affected?	Normal (½ mark)	Depleted (½ mark)
State one other common pathological appearance that is characteristic of the disease	Granulomas (½ mark) Fibrosis (½ mark) Fistulae (½ mark) Sinus formation (½ mark)	Crypt abscesses (neutrophil accumulation, sterile) (½ mark) Pseudopolyps (½ mark)

LEARNING POINT

Inflammatory bowel disease is more common in the western world and has a peak incidence between 20 and 40 years. The aetiology is unknown but environmental factors probably trigger a response in a genetically predisposed individual.

Crohn's disease

Commonest site is terminal ileum. Abdominal pain, malabsorption and weight loss are common. If the colon is involved, diarrhoea and bleeding occur. In perianal disease, skin tags, fissures, abscesses and fistulae are common. Macroscopically, deep ulcers and fissures are visible. This is known as a cobblestone appearance.

Ulcerative colitis

Affects only rectum and colon. The disease process is continuous through the colon and rectum. Diarrhoea with blood and mucus is common. Macroscopically the mucosa appears red and bleeds easily. Ulcers and pseudopolyps may be visible in severe disease (regenerating mucosa).

Mr McDonald is commenced on corticosteroids to control the initial episode of IBD. He remains well.

Q **8. Which colonic pathology can develop in patients who have long-standing inflammatory bowel disease, particularly ulcerative colitis?** *1 mark*

A Colonic cancer /colonic adenocarcinoma.

📖 BIBLIOGRAPHY

Ganong W F. 2005. *Review of Medical Physiology*, 22nd edn. New York: McGraw-Hill Medical.

Guyton A C, Hall J E. 2000. *Textbook of Medical Physiology*, 10th edn. Philadelphia: WB Saunders Co.

Kumar P, Clark M. 2005. *Clinical Medicine*, 6th edn. Edinburgh: Elsevier Saunders.

Kumar V, Cotran R, Robbins S. 2003. *Basic Pathology*, 7th edn. London: WB Saunders.

MacSween R N M, Whaley K. 1992. *Muir's Textbook of Pathology*, 13th edn. London: Arnold.

[a]Georg Meissner (1829–1905), a German anatomist and physiologist. In 1862, he described the submucosal nervous plexus in the intestine. He also described the tactile end-organs in the skin, Meissner's corpuscles.

[b]Leopold Auerbach (1828–1897), German anatomist and neurophysiologist. He described the intrinsic innervation of the bowel and the myenteric plexus using specific stains and light microscopy.

[c]Burrill Bernard Crohn (1884–1983), American gastroenterologist. Crohn's disease is named after him although it had been described independently in 1904 by Polish surgeon Antoni Lesniowski.

GASTROENTEROLOGY
3. PAINLESS JAUNDICE

Mr McMurdo is a 57-year-old man who presents because he has become jaundiced. He has lost weight over the last few weeks and recently has been feeling tired and somewhat depressed. He had previously been in good health. On abdominal examination, there is no tenderness but the fundus of the gallbladder is palpable.

Q 1. What is the surface marking for the fundus of the gallbladder?   *1 mark*

A The surface marking of the fundus of the gallbladder is where the right side of the rectus abdominis muscle meets the costal margin.

> ## 📁 LEARNING POINT
>
> Students and surgeons often say it is at the tip of the 9th costal cartilage. While this is true, it is useless information because costal cartilages cannot be readily distinguished as they join together.

2. In surgery, what is Courvoisier's Law?   *1 mark*

A Courvoisier's Law[a] states that painless jaundice and a palpable gallbladder are rarely due to gallstones (1 mark), ie due to tumour or other pathology.

You also notice that Mr McMurdo has a number of scratch marks on his arms and legs. He volunteers that he has an itch which is extremely distressing and complains that it keeps him awake at night.

Q 3(a). Explain the likely cause of his itch. *1 mark*

A Itch in obstructive jaundice is due to the deposition of bile salts in the skin.

Q 3(b). Cholestyramine is used to treat this itch. Briefly outline its mechanism of action. *1 mark*

A The most useful treatment is cholestyramine (colestyramine or 'colestipol'), an anion exchange resin (½ mark). It acts by binding to bile acids in the small intestine and blocking their reabsorption, thus inhibiting the enterohepatic recirculation (½ mark).

📁 LEARNING POINT

Anion exchange resins also have a role in lipid-lowering therapy. By inhibiting the enterohepatic recycling of bile acids, anion exchange resins increase the metabolism of endogenous cholesterol in the liver to the primary bile acids cholic acid and chenodeoxycholic acid. This then leads to an increased expression of low-density lipoprotein (LDL) receptors on liver cells causing increased LDL removal from the blood and so a reduced LDL-cholesterol level. These drugs can be used in addition to statin therapy in individuals who have had a sub-optimal response to the statin, eg in heterozygous familial hypercholesterolaemia. These drugs are not absorbed and so systemic side-effects are rare but they can, however, cause a number of gastrointestinal side-effects, eg bloating, nausea and diarrhoea.

Q 3(c). Name two other medications that might also help. *1 mark*

A Rifampicin (½ mark) and ursodeoxycholic acid (UDCA) (½ mark) may also be helpful for this type of itch.

Blood tests indicate the presence of obstructive jaundice.

Tests are also carried out to investigate the synthetic function of Mr McMurdo's liver.

Q 4. Complete this table to indicate and explain the abnormal test result expected.

4 marks

Test used	Abnormality expected	Brief explanation outlining why this would occur
Prothrombin time (PT)	Prolonged (1 mark)	The liver is the site of clotting factor synthesis (1 mark). All the clotting factors except factor VIII are made within the liver. The vitamin-K- dependent factors (II, VII, IX and X) may be deficient due to malabsorption of vitamin K.
Albumin	Decreased (1 mark)	This occurs due to reduced synthetic function of the liver. Albumin is synthesised only in the liver (1 mark) and about 10 g is produced each day.

📁 LEARNING POINT

Prothrombin time is predominantly a measure of the extrinsic clotting cascade. It may be prolonged by causes other than impaired liver function, eg vitamin K malabsorption, warfarin administration and disseminated intravascular coagulopathy (DIC). If the prolonged prothrombin time is due to synthetic dysfunction of the liver, vitamin K is administered intramuscularly but will not completely correct it.

During the history, Mr McMurdo said he has lost 7 kg in weight over the past 6 months. More recently he has also noticed a change in his bowel habit. He complains of pale, whitish, greasy stools that are often difficult to flush away (steatorrhea).

Q 5. Explain why his stools are white.

1 mark

A Obstructed bile duct.

Q **6. Name two substances formed from bile pigments that give the stools their characteristic colour.** *2 marks*

A Urobilinogen (1 mark) and stercobilinogen (1 mark).

Mr McMurdo also complains of darkened urine.

Q **7. What two biochemical abnormalities in the urine are seen in this type of jaundice?** *2 marks*

A Low/absent urobilinogen (1 mark) and high urinary bilirubin (1 mark).

Due to your clinical suspicions you refer Mr McMurdo urgently for endoscopic retrograde cholangiopancreatography (ERCP). At ERCP a protrusion was seen at the head of the pancreas and biopsy samples were taken.

Q **8. To which region of the peritoneal cavity is the pancreas particularly related?** *1 mark*

A The lesser sac (omental bursa).

Q **9. How is a pancreatic mass most likely to cause jaundice?** *3 marks*

A The common bile duct (1 mark) runs posterior to or is embedded within (1 mark) the head (1 mark) of the pancreas.

Q **10. Label this diagram of the liver and biliary tree (Figure 3.5).** *6 marks*

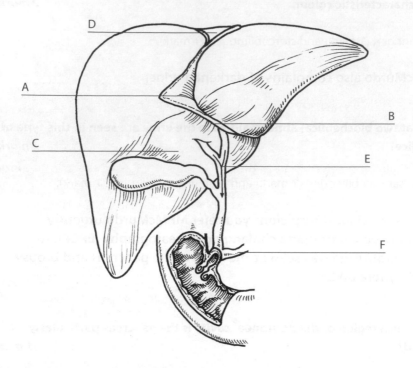

Figure 3.5: The liver and biliary tree.

A 1 mark for each of the following:

A Falciform ligament.

B Round ligament (Ligamentum teres).

C Quadrate lobe.

D Bare area.

E Common hepatic duct.

F Pancreatic duct.

Later in the day of his ERCP, Mr McMurdo started to complain of severe epigastric pain that radiated through to his back.

Q **11. What is the likely cause of this pain?** *1 mark*

A Acute pancreatitis.

 LEARNING POINT

Acute pancreatitis is one of the most common complications of ERCP.

Q **12. Explain Mr McMurdo's back pain.** *1 mark*

A The pancreas is a retroperitoneal organ (½ mark) and so leakage of the inflammatory exudate into the retroperitoneal space and lesser sac causes irritation of retroperitoneal and peritoneal sensory nerve endings (½ mark) and so produces the characteristic intense back pain.

On examination Mr McMurdo has a bluish discoloration of his umbilicus and his flanks.

Q **13. Name these two clinical signs.** *1 mark*

- Cullen's[b] sign (½ mark) – umbilical discoloration (this can also be seen in ruptured ectopic pregnancy).

- Grey Turner's[c] sign (½ mark) – flank discoloration.

As a result of this complication, Mr McMurdo is admitted to ITU and, fortunately, soon recovers from it. The histology from his biopsy samples returns, showing an adenocarcinoma of the pancreas. Further staging indicates that the tumour is resectable. The most common curative operation carried out for head of pancreas is a Whipple's procedure, which involves the en bloc excision of the distal two-thirds of the stomach, distal common bile duct, gallbladder, head of the pancreas and duodenum.

Due to the removal of such a large proportion of the pancreas, malabsorption is likely to occur.

Q **14. The pancreolauryl test can be used to assess exocrine pancreatic function. Briefly outline how this test works.**   *3 marks*

A Any six of the following:

A The test involves the oral administration (½ mark) of fluorescein dilaurate (½ mark), which is poorly absorbed by the gut (½ mark). Pancreatic esterase (½ mark) converts fluorescein dilaurate to fluorescein (½ mark), which is readily absorbed by the gut (½ mark). Once absorbed the fluorescein is excreted in the urine (½ mark). Thus, the presence of fluorescein in the urine is a measure of pancreatic function (½ mark).

📁 LEARNING POINT

Carcinoma of the head of pancreas is more common in men and usually presents between the ages of 50 and 60. The majority of the tumours arise in the head of the pancreas and will present early with obstructive jaundice in association with weight loss. The remainder of the tumours occur in the neck, body and tail and they commonly present late with vague symptoms including epigastric pain, weight loss and anorexia. Examination reveals a thin, cachetic individual who is jaundiced. There may be a palpable gallbladder in the presence of jaundice (Courvoisier's Sign) or even a palpable abdominal mass. Investigations reveal an obstructive picture with a raised alkaline phosphatase, bilirubin and γ-glutamyl transferase. ERCP with biopsy samples is the investigation of choice and therapeutic stenting may be carried out to allow bile drainage. Serological testing with CA 19-9 may be useful and is often raised in pancreatic carcinoma. Unfortunately pancreatic carcinoma has a very bleak prognosis with mean survival time from diagnosis of between 3 and 6 months.

BIBLIOGRAPHY

Boon NA, Colledge NR, Walker BR, Hunter JAA. 2006. *Davidson's Principles and Practices of Medicine*, 20th edn. Edinburgh: Elsevier Churchill Livingstone.

Hempfling W, Dilger K, Beuers U. 2003. Systematic review: ursodeoxycholic acid – adverse effects and drug interactions. *Alimentary Pharmacology and Therapeutics*, **18**, 963–973.

Kumar P, Clark M. 2005. *Clinical Medicine*, 6th edn. Edinburgh: Elsevier Saunders.

Provan D, Krentz A. 2002. *Oxford Handbook of Clinical and Laboratory Investigation*. Oxford: Oxford University Press.

Smith ME, Morton DG. 2001. *The Digestive System*. Edinburgh: Churchill Livingstone.

Twycross R, Greaves MW, Handwerker H, Jones EA, Libretto SE, Szepietowski JC, Zylicz Z. 2003. Itch: scratching more than the surface. *Quarterly Journal of Medicine*, **96**, 7–23.

[a]Ludwig Courvoisier (1843–1918), Swiss surgeon who became Professor of Surgery at the University of Basle. Courvoisier's Law was first stated in a book published by him in 1890 on the pathology and surgery of the gall bladder.

[h]Thomas S. Cullen (1868–1953), Canadian obstetrician and gynaecologist who first described the sign of bruising around the umbilicus in ruptured ectopic pregnancy in 1916.

[c]George Grey Turner (1877–1951), English surgeon who first described discoloration of the flanks in pancreatitis. As a young surgeon, he travelled widely and was received by the Pope, Mussolini, the King of Italy and King Alfonso of Spain. He was Professor of Surgery at Newcastle and later at the Postgraduate Medical School, Hammersmith.

GASTROENTEROLOGY

GASTROENTEROLOGY
4. LIVER DISEASE

Mr Fraser is a 56-year-old man who presents to his GP with a 4-day history of worsening yellow discoloration of his skin and eyes. He is thin, has lost his appetite and complains of nausea, tiredness and upper abdominal discomfort especially on the right side. On examination he is markedly jaundiced and you find that he has an enlarged liver, ascites and gynaecomastia, but no spleen is palpable.

Q **1. Define ascites.**   *1 mark*

A Ascites is the accumulation of free fluid in the peritoneal cavity.

Q **2. Give three conditions that might give rise to ascites.**   *1½ marks*

A **Chronic liver disease**   *½ mark*

Chronic heart disease   *½ mark*

Abdominal malignancy   *½ mark*

LEARNING POINT

There are a number of theories about the development of the sodium and water retention seen in ascites:

- Overflow theory: that a primary renal retention of sodium and water leads to an increased blood volume and 'spillage' of excess fluid into the peritoneal space.
- Underfilling theory: that leakage of fluid into the peritoneal cavity results in a compensatory renal retention of sodium and water.
- Vasodilation theory: that splanchnic vasodilatation causes a reduction in effective circulating blood volume, which leads to activation of the renin–angiotensin system resulting in sodium and water retention. This appears to be the most important pathogenic factor.

Ascitic fluid may be an exudate or a transudate. Analysis may help with diagnosis. Albumin levels significantly below serum levels suggest a transudate.

Q 3. Explain the pathophysiology of gynaecomastia.　　　*2 marks*

A Gynaecomastia is due to increased oestrogen levels (1 mark). The increased oestrogen results from a decreased clearance of endogenous oestrogens by the diseased liver (1 mark).

 LEARNING POINT

The reduced clearance of endogenous oestrogens combined with reduced hepatic synthesis of steroid-hormone-binding globulin results in tissues receiving higher than normal concentrations of oestrogens. In addition a longer half-life of androgens allows a greater degree of peripheral aromatisation (conversion to oestrogens by, eg adipose tissue, hair follicles) further increasing oestrogen-like effects.

GASTROENTEROLOGY

Q **4. In the presence of portal hypertension the spleen may be enlarged. Why is this?** *1 mark*

A The splenic vein is a tributary of the portal vein (½ mark). The portal venous system does not contain valves (½ mark) so in portal hypertension the spleen becomes congested and enlarged.

Q **5. Supply the missing words.** *2 marks*

Q **2 marks in total: ½ mark for each:**

A The normal spleen lies in the left *hypochondriac* region of the abdomen. The spleen lies at the level of the *9th* to the 11th ribs. A normal spleen lies posterior to the mid-axillary line and is separated from the left lung by the *diaphragm* covered superiorly by the *pleura* and inferiorly by the peritoneum.

As you examine Mr Fraser further, you begin to think about the histological structure of the liver.

Q **6. In the diagram (Figure 3.6) below identify unit of liver A and unit of liver structure B. Identify features C, D and E.** *5 marks*

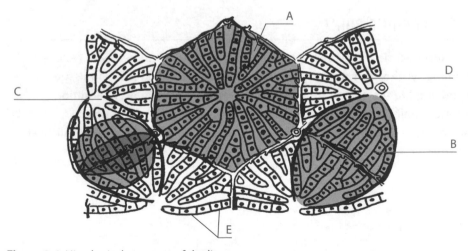

Figure 3.6: Histological structure of the liver.

A A – Classical lobule

B – Liver acinus

C – Central vein

D – Liver sinusoid

E – Hepatocytes/hepatocyte plates

Q **7. Where are the portal tracts situated?** *1 mark*

A At the corners of the classical lobules.

Q **8. Name the three tubular structures found in a portal tract.** *1 mark*

A Branches of the hepatic artery, portal vein and bile ductule (1 mark – must get all three).

 LEARNING POINT

The branches of the hepatic artery and the portal vein and the bile ductule are collectively known as the portal triad. The portal tracts also contain lymphatics.

Q **9. Give two ways in which the cellular lining of the liver sinusoids is specialised to aid liver function.** *2 marks*

A Endothelium is fenestrated (½ mark) to enhance permeability (½ mark).

A Kupffer cells[a] (½ mark) lie in the endothelial layer and are phagocytic (½ mark).

369

LEARNING POINT

The Kupffer cells have a role in immunity and are part of the mononuclear phagocyte system. They remove aged and damaged erythrocytes, bacteria and antigen–antibody complexes from the circulation. They also produce a variety of cytokines which can act locally or be secreted into the systemic circulation. They are derived from circulating monocytes and essentially act like macrophages.

Q 10. What is the perisinusoidal space (of Disseᵇ) and what function does it assist? *1 mark*

A The space of Disse is the region between hepatocytes and the sinusoid lining (½ mark). It contains microvilli from the non-canalicular surfaces of hepatocytes. Its presence increases the interface between hepatocytes and fluid that passes from/to the sinusoid lumen via the fenestrations. It thus facilitates exchange of substances between the blood and the hepatocytes (½ mark).

Upon further questioning Mr Fraser tells you that he is an alcoholic with a prolonged history of excess drinking over about ten years. He has been drinking about 40 units a week with recent binges. You suspect alcoholic liver disease.

Q 11(a). What substance is produced in the first step of alcohol metabolism catalysed by cytoplasmic alcohol dehydrogenase? *1 mark*

A Acetaldehyde.

Q 11(b). Is this metabolic pathway inducible? *1 mark*

A No.

Q 11(c). Which other metabolic pathway is involved in alcohol metabolism? *1 mark*

A The microsomal ethanol oxidising system (MEOS).

Blood results:

Test	GGT (IU/l)	Alkaline phosphatase (U/l)	AST (IU/l)	ALT (IU/l)	Total bilirubin (µmol/l)
Result	148 (11–58)	136 (39–117)	151 (12–40)	72 (5–40)	130 (less than 17)

Q 12(a). Define the type of jaundice. *1 mark*

A Hepatocellular jaundice.

Q 12(b). What is the significance of each of the following observations?

Q i. Markedly raised levels of aspartate transaminase and alanine transaminase? *½ mark*

A Hepatocyte damage (½ mark)

🗁 LEARNING POINT

In alcoholic hepatitis the AST:ALT ratio is often greater than 2.

Q ii. Markedly elevated gamma-glutamyl transferase? *½ mark*

A Alcohol-related disease.

Q iii. Elevated level of alkaline phosphatase? *½ mark*

A Obstruction of bile ductules because of the inflammation of the liver parenchyma.

A full blood count has also been carried out and a macrocytic anaemia with a neurophilia is reported.

Q 13. What are the two most likely explanations for the macrocytosis? *1 mark*

A Alcohol (½ mark) – this is thought to be due to the suppressant effect that alcohol has on the bone marrow *and* folic acid deficiency (½ mark).

Q 14. Put the following features of alcoholic liver disease in order of most likely progression. *1 mark*

A Steatosis – Alcoholic hepatitis – Cirrhosis – Hepatocellular carcinoma (1 mark – must get all four in correct order).

A liver biopsy is carried out on Mr Fraser. It confirms your clinical suspicion that he has alcoholic hepatitis.

Q 15. Give four characteristic features of alcoholic hepatitis as seen on light microscopy of the biopsy specimen. *4 marks*

A Any 4 of the following, 4 marks in total:

- Presence of fatty change (1 mark).
- Neutrophil infiltrate (1 mark).
- Hepatocyte ballooning/necrosis (1 mark).
- Mallory bodies (alcoholic hyaline) (1 mark).
- Early deposition of fibrous tissue (1 mark).

The biopsy and radiological imaging suggest that Mr Fraser's liver disease has not progressed to cirrhosis.

Q 16. Define cirrhosis. *1 mark*

A Any of the points below up to a maximum of 1 mark:

A Cirrhosis is a diffuse process where there is repeated hepatocyte destruction (½ mark) followed by regeneration to replace lost cells (½ mark). There is also deposition of collagenous tissue (scarring) (½ mark). The combination of nodules of regenerated hepatocytes separated by scar tissue is known as cirrhosis (½ mark).

 LEARNING POINT

Cirrhosis results in impairment of liver function and destruction of the normal liver architecture, which ultimately results in portal hypertension.

Grossly and histologically two types of cirrhosis are often described:
- **Micronodular cirrhosis, characterised by uniform small nodules usually less than 3 mm in diameter. This is the sub-type commonly seen in alcoholic cirrhosis.**
- **Macronodular cirrhosis in which larger nodules are seen that may be up to about 2 cm in diameter. This is often seen following chronic hepatitis B infection.**

However, a mixed picture can occur.

 BIBLIOGRAPHY

Boon N A, Colledge N R, Walker B R, Hunter J A A. 2006. *Davidson's Principles and Practice of Medicine*, 20th edn. Edinburgh: Elsevier Churchill Livingstone.

Fawcett D W. 1994. *A Textbook of Histology*. New York: Chapman and Hall.

Kumar P, Clark M. 2005. *Clinical Medicine*, 6th edn. Edinburgh: Elsevier Saunders.

McPhee S J, Ganong W F. 2006. *Pathophysiology of Disease*, 5th edn. New York: Lange Medical Books/McGraw-Hill.

Provan D, Krentz A. 2002. *Oxford Handbook of Clinical and Laboratory Investigation*. Oxford: Oxford University Press.

Smith M E, Morton D G. 2001. *The Digestive System*. Edinburgh: Churchill Livingstone.

GASTROENTEROLOGY

Sorbi D, Boynton J, Lindor K D. 1999. The ratio of aspartate aminotransferase to alanine aminotransferase: potential value in differentiating nonalcoholic steatohepatitis from alcoholic liver disease. *Am J Gastroenterol*, **94**, 1018–1022.

[a]Karl Wilhelm von Kupffer (1829–1902), German anatomist born in Kurland, now part of Latvia. He described the Kupffer cells in 1876 and thought they were endothelial cells. They were discovered to be macrophages by Tadeusz Browicz in 1898.

[b]Joseph Disse (1852–1912), German anatomist who discovered the perisinusoidal space. He had wide interests in experimental pathology including the development of the paranasal sinuses and the vascular system of the chick.

GASTROENTEROLOGY
5. GASTRO-OESOPHAGEAL REFLUX DISEASE

Mr Anderson is a 57-year-old businessman who smokes 15 cigarettes per day and typically has his main meal in the later evening along with a glass of wine. He presents to his GP with heartburn, belching and waterbrash. His GP suspects that he is suffering from gastro-oesophageal reflux disease.

Q **1. Where does the pharynx become continuous with the oesophagus?** *1 mark*

A At the lower limit of the larynx (cricoid cartilage) or at the level of C6 vertebra.

Q **2. In which regions of the mediastinum does the oesophagus lie?** *1 mark*

A The oesophagus passes through the superior and posterior parts of the mediastinum (must get both parts of the mediastinum to get 1 mark).

Q **3. Where does the oesophagus enter the abdominal cavity?** *1 mark*

A It passes through the right crus (½ mark) of the diaphragm. This occurs slightly to the left of the midline (½ mark) or at the level of T10 vertebra (½ mark).

Q **4. What anatomical and physiological arrangements protect against gastro-oesophageal reflux?** *2 marks*

A Any four of the following (½ mark each):

- Lower oesophageal (cardiac) sphincter.

- The angle between the lower oesophagus and the fundus of the stomach.

- Mucosal rosette formed by folds of mucosa at the gastro-oesophageal junction.

- The crura of the diaphragm surrounding the oesophagus.

- Oesophageal peristalsis.

- Gastric peristalsis.

📁 **LEARNING POINT**

The lower oesophageal sphincter refers to the smooth muscle of the muscularis externa at the oesophagogastric junction. The smooth muscle at this site is no thicker than in adjacent regions.

Factors predisposing to reflux include:

Defective lower oesophageal sphincter function. This can be secondary to smoking, fatty meals, delayed gastric emptying or following sphincter surgery in achalasia.

Increased intra-abdominal pressure. This may be secondary to tight-fitting clothes, obesity, large meals, pregnancy, ascites or an abdominal or pelvic mass.

Drugs, eg tricyclic antidepressants and anticholinergics.

Because of his age, Mr Anderson was referred for further investigation. Upper GI endoscopy and barium swallow were carried out. Barium swallow revealed a sliding hiatus hernia.

Q 5. What is a hiatus hernia?   *1 mark*

A A hiatus hernia is where the upper part of the stomach protrudes through the diaphragm into the thoracic cavity.

Q 6. Describe the difference between a sliding hiatus hernia and a rolling hiatus hernia.   *2 marks*

A A sliding hiatus hernia is where the gastro-oesophageal junction slides up into the chest (1 mark). A rolling (para-oesophageal) hernia is where the gastric fundus protrudes up alongside the oesophagus, usually to its left (1 mark).

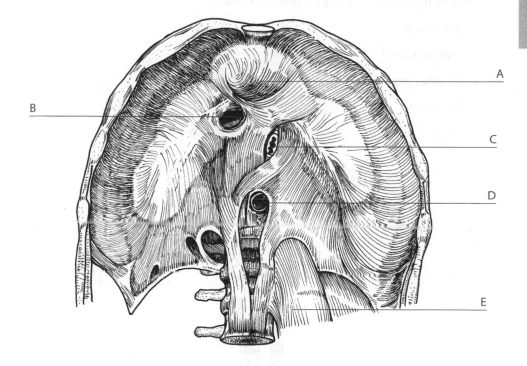

Figure 3.7: The diaphragm.

Q **7. On the above drawing of the diaphragm (Figure 3.7), identify A–E.** *5 marks*

A – Central tendon

B – Inferior vena cava

C – Oesophagus

D – Aorta

E – Psoas major muscle

Q **8. Label A–E on the following diagram (Figure 3.8).** *2½ marks*

Choose from the following (½ mark for each):

- **Chief cells.**

- **Gastric gland.**

- **Mucous neck cells.**

- **Gastric pit.**

- **Parietal cells.**

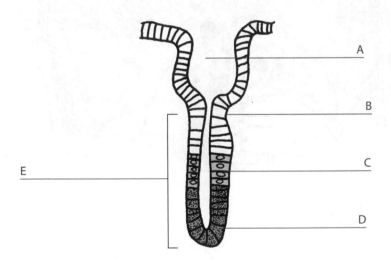

Figure 3.8: Epithelial cells of the stomach

A A – Gastric pit.

B – Mucous neck cells.

C – Parietal cells.

D – Chief cells.

E – Gastric gland.

Q 9. What type of cell is found on the mucosal surface of the stomach lumen? *½ mark*

A Surface mucous cells.

 LEARNING POINT

In these cells the mucus does not form goblets.

Q 10. Which of the cell types in the gastric mucosa secretes hydrochloric acid? *1 mark*

A Parietal cell.

Q 11. Which cell type in the gastric mucosa secretes pepsinogen? *1 mark*

A Chief cell.

Q 12. Which cell type in the gastric mucosa secretes intrinsic factor? *1 mark*

A Parietal cell.

Q 13. Why is intrinsic factor important? *1 mark*

A It binds to vitamin B_{12} (½ mark) and allows it to be absorbed from the ileum (½ mark).

Q 14(a). Describe the mechanism of acid secretion in the stomach. *2 marks*

A Any four of the following (½ mark each):

- Parietal cells are rich in carbonic anhydrase.

- $CO_2 + H_2O \rightarrow H_2CO_3 \rightarrow H^+ + HCO_3^-$.

- Above reaction catalysed by carbonic anhydrase.

- H^+ is pumped into the lumen of the stomach via primary H^+/K^+ ATP-ases (proton pumps) at the luminal membrane.

- HCO_3 is secreted at the basolateral membrane in exchange for chloride ions.

- Acid is released into the intracellular canaliculus of the parietal cell.

Q 14(b). Name four mediators that augment acid secretion. *2 marks*

A Any two of (½ mark each):

- Histamine.

- Acetylcholine.

- Gastrin.

- Somatostatin.

During the upper GI endoscopy, the oesophagogastric junction was visualised. It revealed gastro-oesophageal reflux disease (GORD) with no complications.

Q 15. What type of epithelium lines the oesophagus? *1 mark*

A Stratified squamous (½ mark) non-keratinised (½ mark) epithelium.

The endoscopy report also mentioned that there was no evidence of 'the metaplastic changes of Barrett's oesophagus'.

Q 16. What is 'metaplasia'? *1 mark*

A Metaplasia is a change in the cells from one form to another.

Q 17. What is the clinical significance of Barrett's oesophagus? *1 mark*

A Its presence is understood to increase the risk of oesophageal cancer.

It is decided that Mr Anderson should be managed non-surgically with regular follow-up. You advise him on lifestyle changes, including cessation of smoking, limitation of large meals and eating near bedtime, and raising the head of the bed at night. You also prescribe some drugs.

Q 18. Name three drugs that can be used to manage a patient with gastro-oesophageal reflux disease and describe their mechanisms of action. *3 marks*

A Any three of the following drugs and their mechanisms:

Drug	Mechanism of action
Omeprazole (½ mark) Other examples of proton pump inhibitors include lansoprazole, pantoprazole	Proton pump inhibitor (½ mark)
Cimetidine (½ mark) Other examples of H_2-receptor antagonists include ranitidine and famotidine	H_2-receptor antagonist (½ mark)
Gaviscon (½ mark)	Alginate: forms a 'raft' that floats on the surface of stomach contents to reduce reflux (½ mark)
Aluminium hydroxide (½ mark) Another antacid is magnesium carbonate	Aluminium hydroxide is an antacid which act by binding to free H^+ ions (½ mark)
Metoclopramide (½ mark)	Prokinetic drug: may improve gastro-oesophageal sphincter function and accelerate gastric emptying (½ mark)

GASTROENTEROLOGY

BIBLIOGRAPHY

Kumar P, Clark M. 2005. *Clinical Medicine*, 6th edn. Edinburgh: Elsevier Saunders.

Standring S. 2005. *Gray's Anatomy*, 39th edn. Edinburgh: Elsevier Churchill Livingstone.

Widmaier EP, Raff H, Strang KT. 2006. *Vander's Human Physiology: the Mechanisms of Body Function*, 10th edn. Boston: McGraw Hill.

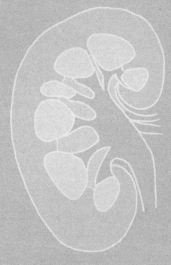

NEPHROLOGY CASE:
ANSWERS

NEPHROLOGY
1. CHRONIC RENAL FAILURE

Mr Shilliday is a pleasant 72-year-old man who comes to see you at the GP surgery because of a 2-month history of non-specific symptoms that include increasing tiredness, loss of appetite and generally feeling not quite himself. His skin is very itchy. You last saw him 1 year ago when he was very well.

The practice nurse takes a blood sample to check his liver function tests, his urea and electrolytes and his full blood count. You ask him to return in 48 hours.

These investigations reveal the following results:

FBC:
- **Haemoglobin – 7 (13–18 g/dl)**
- **MCV – 83 (76–96 fl)**
- **WCC – 8 [(4–11)×10⁹/l]**
- **Platelets – 250 [(150–400)× 10⁹/l]**

U&Es:

- Na – 129 (135–145 mmol/l)
- K – 5.1 (3.5–5 mmol/l)
- Urea – 60 (2.5–6.7 mmol/l)
- Creatinine – 999 (70–150 μmol/l)
- Glucose – 5 (3.5–5.5 mmol/l)
- Ca – 1.6 (2.05–2.6 mmol/l)
- PO_4^{2-} – 3.5 (0.8–1.4 mmol/l)

LFTs
- Albumin – 15 (35–50 g/l)
- Aspartate aminotransferase (AST) – 30 (3–35 iu/l)
- Alanine aminotransferase (ALT) – 20 (3–35 iu/l)
- Alkaline phosphatase – 300 (30–35 iu/l)

From these results you suspect that he has chronic renal failure (CRF).

Q 1. List six results, which are strongly in keeping with this diagnosis, apart from raised serum creatinine and hypocalcaemia. *3 marks*

A ½ mark each for:

- High urea

- Anaemia

- Mild hyperkalaemia (must be mild – if it was very high this would mean acute renal failure)

- Hyperphosphataemia

- Hypoalbuminaemia

- High alkaline phosphatase

📁 LEARNING POINTS

Chronic renal failure is defined as a loss of renal function, which is slowly progressive, often longstanding and usually associated with irreversible structural damage. The major causes vary with age. In Scotland in a man of this age the commonest cause is related to widespread vascular disease and atheroma. An approximately equal number are reported as being of unknown cause. Chronic glomerulonephritis, chronic interstitial nephritis and diabetes mellitus have much lower incidence. This should be compared to the causes found in those less than 45 years of age, where the commonest causes are chronic infection, interstitial nephritis, congenital disease, glomerulonephritis and diabetes mellitus.

For more information see Scottish Renal Registry.

You ask the medical student who has been placed with you what she thinks of the results. Using her knowledge of renal physiology you ask her to explain the following.

Q 2. Why is serum creatinine a good marker of glomerular filtration rate? *2 marks*

A Total of 2 marks from the following:

NEPHROLOGY

A Creatinine is produced from skeletal muscle at a relatively steady rate (½ mark). It is freely filtered at the glomeruli (½ mark) and then neither secreted into nor reabsorbed from the tubular filtrate to any significant degree (½ mark). Under those circumstances the amount filtered per unit time (GFR × plasma concentration) will equal the amount excreted in the same time (urine concentration × urine flow rate) (½ mark). GFR thus equals urine concentration × urine flow rate/plasma concentration of creatinine (½ mark).

📂 LEARNING POINTS

An important consequence of this relationship is that the concentration of creatinine in the blood is directionally proportional to the total glomerular filtration rate. Thus the concentration of serum creatinine doubles with each 50% reduction in GFR.

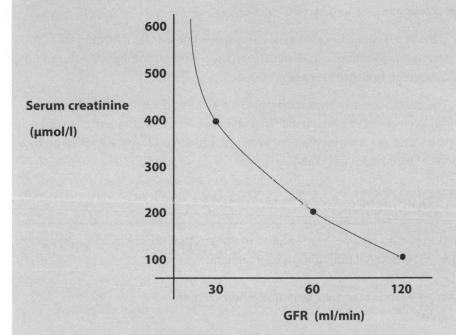

For example, in a patient with stable CRF, a serum creatinine concentration of 200 μmol/l tells us that the patient has lost approximately half of their overall normal renal function.

It is apparent from the results of his FBC that Mr Shilliday has a normocytic, normochromic anaemia.

Q **3. Explain how this has come about.** *2 marks*

A Fall in production of erythropoietin (EPO) (½ mark) by the damaged kidneys (½ mark). This hormone is made in the renal tubular cells in response to hypoxia (½ mark) Normally this will ensure appropriate rates of erythropoiesis in red bone marrow. In CRF insufficient EPO is made resulting in the production of a reduced number of erythrocytes of normal size and haemoglobin content (½ mark).

Q **4. Explain the origin of the hypocalcaemia.** *2 marks*

A Hypocalcaemia is caused by two mechanisms:

1. Defective renal hydroxylation of 25-hydroxycholecalciferol leading to reduced production of 1,25-dihydroxycholecalciferol and hence reduced Ca absorption from gut (1 mark).

2. The consequence of hyperphosphataemia due to a fall in GFR and hence a fall in renal loss of phosphate. Since the product of calcium and phosphate in the blood is kept within a narrow range, a rise in phosphate is followed by a fall in blood calcium (1 mark).

🗁 LEARNING POINT

The kidney is a very important endocrine organ that produces a number of important hormonal functions, which include:
- EPO
- Active vitamin D or 1,25-dihydroxycholecalciferol
- Renin

Patients with end-stage CRF can now be given EPO and active vitamin D, resulting in a vast improvement in their symptoms due to chronic anaemia and metabolic bone disease.

Since she has answered so well you try some basic anatomy questions!

Q 5. Name the structures indicated in the diagram below (Figure 4.1). *3 marks*

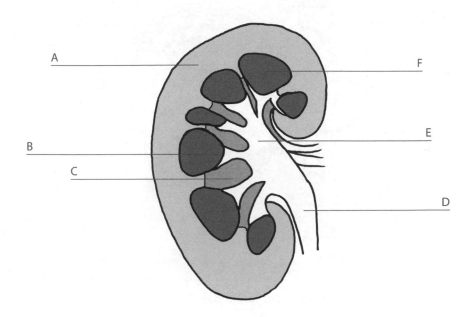

Figure 4.1: The kidney.

A ½ mark for each of following:

A –Renal cortex

B – Renal papilla

C –Renal sinus

D –Renal pelvis

E – Major calyx

F – Renal pyramid

Q **6. Name structures A–D on the diagram (Figure 4.2) shown below of a normal glomerulus.** *4 marks*

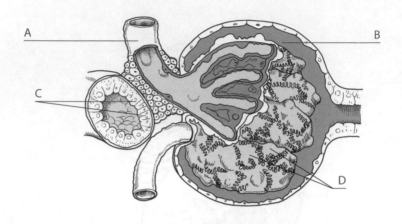

Figure 4.2: The normal glomerulus.

A The four items to name (1 mark each) would be:

A   Afferent arteriole

B   Bowman's space

C   Macula densa

D   Podocytes

Q 7. List three other tests, apart from blood tests, which you could now organise yourself in order to determine the cause of Mr Shilliday's CRF.   *3 marks*

A

Test	Mark	Finding suggestive of CRF	Mark
Blood pressure lying and standing	½	Significantly raised	½
Urinalysis	½	Microalbuminaemia or frank proteinuria Glycosuria Haematuria\	½
Abdominal ultrasound	½	Two small shrunken kidneys with or without longstanding obstruction	½

Not acceptable – intravenous pyelogram (IVP), bone radiology, BM stix° (glycosuria picked up on Dipstix).

In view of his advanced CRF, however, you decide to refer Mr Shilliday as soon as possible to the local renal unit to be looked after by the renal physicians. He tells you that he has been suffering from some 'aches and pains' in the last couple of months. You suspect this is most likely due to renal osteodystrophy.

Q 8. What is meant by renal osteodystrophy?   *1 mark*

A Renal osteodystrophy is bone disease due to a combination of disturbed vitamin D metabolism and secondary hyperparathyroidism (½ mark) found in patients with long standing CRF (½ mark).

📁 LEARNING POINT

Renal osteodystrophy is a term that encompasses the variety of bone disease that develops in chronic renal failure. This is caused by disturbed vitamin D metabolism and secondary hyperparathyroidism with raised serum alkaline phosphatase.

This results clinically as bone pain and fracture.

Q 9. Explain with the aid of a diagram (Figure 4.3) the metabolism of vitamin D. *4 marks*

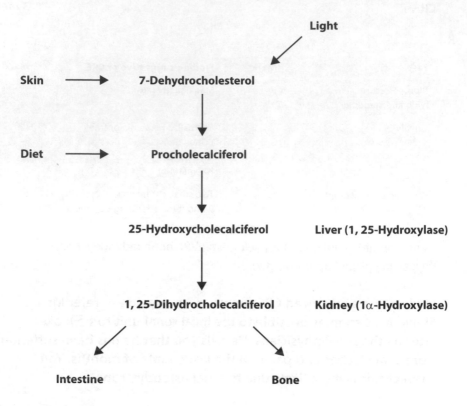

Figure 4.3: The metabolism of vitamin D.

At the local renal unit, biochemical investigation is carried out, which shows that Mr Shilliday has multiple myeloma, a malignant condition of red bone marrow. This is likely to be the cause his renal failure.

Q 10. Name the areas of the body where red bone marrow is found in the adult. *2 marks*

A Red bone marrow is found in the cancellous bone of the axial skeleton (1 mark). These include the sternum, vertebrae, ribs, hip bones, clavicles and skull vault (½ mark for each one cited, max 2 marks).

🗀 LEARNING POINT

In juveniles red marrow is found in long bones of the limbs but by the time adulthood is reached the red marrow is largely confined to the axial skeleton.

Q 11. Name the specific abnormality that can be found in the urine in myeloma. *1 mark*

A 'Bence Jones' protein[a]

Q 12. In the table below list three other tests that can be done to confirm the diagnosis of multiple myeloma and list the abnormality found in each. *3 marks*

Test	Mark	Result indicative of myeloma	Mark
Skeletal survey	½	Osteolytic bone lesions	½
Plasma electrophoresis	½	Monoclonal paraprotein	½
Bone marrow aspirate or trephine	½	Excessive plasma cells in bone marrow	½

LEARNING POINT

Multiple myeloma is characterised by three principal features:
- Production of monoclonal paraprotein – a clone of B-lymphocytes in the bone marrow secretes free immunoglobulin light chains
- The small light chains are freely filtered at the glomerulus and form obstructive casts in the tubules, resulting eventually in death of these nephrons
- There are usually numerous lytic bone lesions, causing bone pain

Mr Shilliday died 6 months later at home.

 BIBLIOGRAPHY

Scottish Renal Registry. Available online at http://www.srr.scot.nhs.uk/ and, more specifically, at http://www.srr.scot.nhs.uk/Report2004/SRR_Report_2002_2004.pdf

Horton-Szar D, Harris K. (eds) 2007. *Renal and Urinary Systems. Crash Course*, 3rd edn. London: Mosby.

[a]H. Bence Jones (1814–1873), English physician and skilled chemist who pioneered a scientific approach to clinical problems. First to describe the abnormal protein found in the urine of patients with multiple myeloma. It is characterised by precipitation at 56ºC and re-solution at 100ºC.

NEPHROLOGY

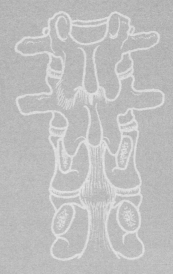

MUSCULOSKELETAL CASES: ANSWERS

MUSCULOSKELETAL
1. MUSCULAR DYSTROPHY

In the week after taking up a new appointment in orthopaedics, you are assisting at the outpatient clinic. One of the patients who attends is 28-year-old Mr Naismith. Before he arrives, you review the case notes. He has Becker's muscular dystrophy. You recall that this is a genetic disorder similar to Duchenne muscular dystrophy with the same form of inheritance. In Becker's muscular dystrophy reduced amounts of dystrophin are produced whereas in Duchenne muscular dystrophy very little is produced.

Q 1. What is the mode of inheritance of Becker's muscular dystrophy? *1 mark*

A X-linked recessive.

Q 2. What is the function of dystrophin? *1 mark*

A Dystrophin connects the cytoskeleton of the muscle fibre with the surrounding extracellular matrix, important in muscle contraction.

Q 3. What is the name given to the basic functional unit of striated muscle? *1 mark*

A Sarcomere.

Q 4. On the following diagram (Figure 5.1) please label the following: *2 marks*

   A band

   I band

   Sarcomere

   Z line

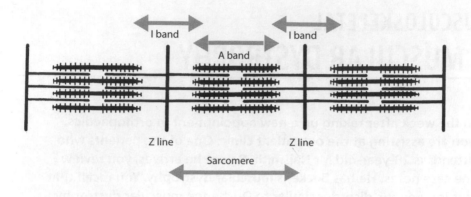

Figure 5.1: Striated muscle.

(2 marks – ½ mark for each.)

Q 5. What composes the thick and thin filaments?   *1 mark*

Thick filament	Myosin (½ mark)	Thin filament	Actin (½ mark)

Contraction of striated muscle is brought about by a mechanism sometimes known as the 'cross-bridge cycle'.

Q 6. What forms the 'cross-bridge'?   *1 mark*

A The myosin head binding to the actin (thin filament).

Q 7. Describe the 'cross-bridge cycle'.   *4 marks*

Cross-bridge forms by myosin head binding to actin filament (1 mark).

Cross-bridge moves, thus sliding the thin filament (1 mark).

Cross-bridge detaches from thin filament (½ mark). ATP binds to myosin (½ mark).

Cross-bridge is energised (by hydrolysis of ATP) (½ mark) so it can reattach to the thin filament and repeat the cycle (½ mark).

LEARNING POINT

The molecular mechanism of contraction is known as the sliding filament mechanism. During shortening of sarcomeres the thick filaments slide past, overlapping thin filaments with no change in the length of either filament. Cross-bridges in the thick filament bind to actin in thin filaments and undergo a conformational change, pulling the thin filament towards the centre of the sarcomere. Cross-bridges repeat their swivelling motion time after time thus leading to large displacements of the filaments. This is known as the cross-bridge cycle.

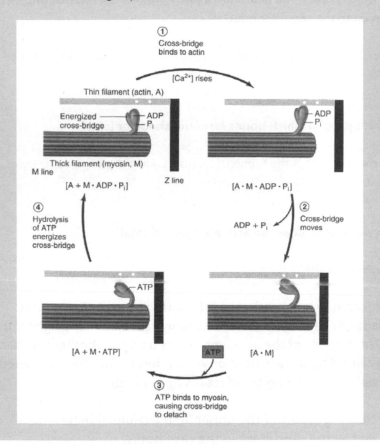

Mr Naismith comes in using crutches. He has been unable to walk unaided for the last 18 months, the dystrophy in his lower limbs having become progressively worse since his late teens. The current problem is that he is on a follow-up visit after a fall four weeks ago. He fell on a step and landed awkwardly striking his right shoulder against a railing. The notes indicated that the shoulder had been quite badly bruised over the acromion but radiology had excluded a fracture or dislocation.

Q **8. Of which bone is the acromion a part? What is the relationship of the acromion to the shoulder joint?** *1 mark*

A The acromion is a projection of the scapula (½ mark) that lies superior to the shoulder joint (½ mark).

Q **9. Which parts of which bones form the shoulder joint?** *2 marks*

A The head (½ mark) of the humerus (½ mark) and the glenoid fossa (½ mark) of the scapula (½ mark).

Q **10. In which joint does the acromion participate?** *1 mark*

A The acromioclavicular joint.

The concern that necessitated follow-up at the clinic was that Mr Naismith had a degree of muscular weakness in his right upper limb. At the time of the accident, it was unclear whether this had been caused by the accident or was an indication that his muscular dystrophy was starting to affect his upper limb.

The following report of the upper limb examination has been recorded by the consultant in the case notes.

- **Right upper limb: General poverty of shoulder movement. Weakness of flexion of the elbow and of supination. Wrist and finger movements** normal. No sensory loss detected. Poor biceps reflex but triceps reflex normal.

- **Left upper limb: No abnormalities detected.**

Q 11. Which muscles flex the elbow? *1 mark*

A Brachialis (½ mark) and biceps (½ mark).

Q 12. Which muscle is the principal supinator? *1 mark*

A Biceps.

📁 LEARNING POINT

Biceps is the main supinator. The supinator muscle only assists with the movement, particularly when the elbow is extended. Biceps is used when opening a bottle (Last and Sinnatamby 1999). Unscrewing and pulling out a cork both use biceps brachii.

You think about the brachial plexus and the peripheral nerves of the upper limb.

Q 13. On the following outline of the brachial plexus (Figure 5.2), label the following. *6 marks*

Ventral ramus of C7

Superior trunk of brachial plexus

Lateral cord of brachial plexus

Median nerve

Radial nerve

Ulnar nerve

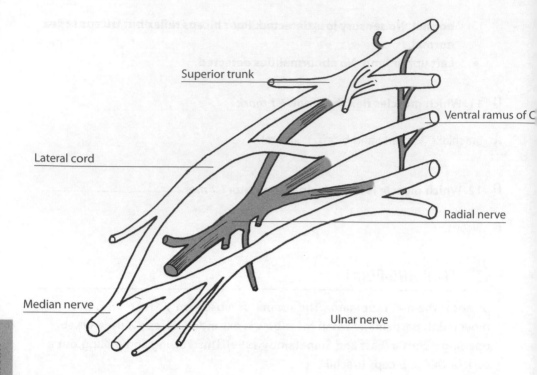

Figure 5.2: Brachial plexus.

Q 14. Do you think the deficits recorded by the consultant suggest neurological damage or progression of the muscular dystrophy? Give reasons for your answer. *6 marks*

A Progression of the muscular dystrophy would be unlikely to conform to a neurological pattern of distribution (1 mark). The description is strongly suggestive of Erb's palsy[a] (1 mark), damage to the C5 and C6 fibres (1 mark) of the superior trunk (1 mark) of the brachial plexus. Neurons from C5 and C6 spinal nerves supply the muscles that move the shoulder joint (1 mark), brachialis and biceps (1 mark).

You examine both upper limbs and find no neurological deficits.

MUSCULOSKELETAL

Q 15. What would be an appropriate medical explanation that you could tell Mr Naismith. *1 mark*

A That the weakness was due to neuropraxia (temporary dysfunction through relatively minor trauma to the nerve fibres).

📖 BIBLIOGRAPHY

Emery A, Muntoni F. 2003. *Duchenne Muscular Dystrophy*, 3rd edn. Oxford: Oxford University Press.

Kumar P, Clark M. 2005. *Clinical Medicine*, 6th edn. Edinburgh: Elsevier Saunders.

Last R J, Sinnatamby C S. 1999. *Last's Anatomy: Regional and Applied (MRCS Study Guides)*. London: Churchill Livingstone.

Nussbaum R L, McInnes R R, Willard H F. 2007. *Genetics in Medicine*, 7th edn. Philadelphia: Saunders.

Standring S. 2005. *Gray's Anatomy*, 39th edn. Edinburgh: Elsevier Churchill Livingstone.

Widmaier E P, Roff H, Strang K T. 2006. *Vander's Human Physiology. The Mechanism of Body Function*, 10th edn. Boston: McGraw Hill.

[a]Wilhelm Heinrich Erb (1840–1921), German neurologist and professor of pathology at Heidelberg. As well as Erb's palsy, he also described myasthenia gravis.

MUSCULOSKELETAL
2. WRIST FRACTURE

Andrew Beattie, a 15-year-old boy, attends the Accident and Emergency Department after a fall at a school rugby match. He had fallen on his outstretched right hand. Movement at the wrist is limited and there is marked tenderness in the anatomical snuffbox. Radiology of the wrist is carried out and the following view obtained (Figure 5.3). The x-ray shows a fracture of the scaphoid bone.

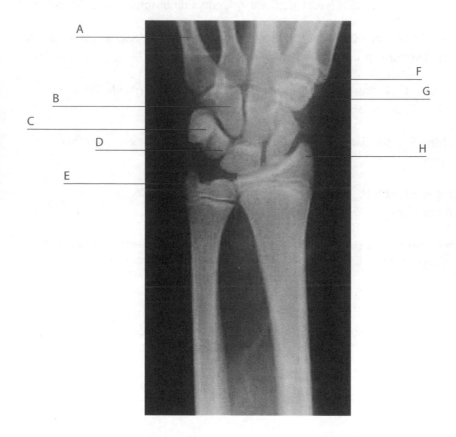

Q **1. Identify the structures labelled A–H in Figure 5.3.**   *4 marks*

A ½ mark for each:

A – Fifth metacarpal

B – Hamate

C – Pisiform

D – Triquetral

E – Styloid process of ulna

F – Epiphysis of first metacarpal

G – Trapezium

H – Styloid process of radius

Q **2. What structures form the medial and lateral boundaries of the anatomical snuffbox?** *1 mark*

Medial boundary	Tendon of extensor pollicis longus (½ mark)
Lateral boundary	Tendon of extensor pollicis brevis (½ mark)

⌐⊐ LEARNING POINT

Tenderness in the anatomical snuffbox is a sign that the scaphoid bone, which lies in the floor of the snuffbox, has been fractured.

Q **3. Andrew's wrist movement was limited. What movements normally occur at the wrist and which are the most restricted?** *4 marks*

A Flexion and extension (1 mark) are the main (1 mark) movements at the wrist.

A Abduction and adduction (1 mark) also occur but are more restricted (1 mark).

MUSCULOSKELETAL

Immobilisation in a plaster splint is required. The plaster is applied as far as the interphalangeal joint of the thumb and the metacarpophalangeal joints of the fingers. This supports the carpus while allowing movement of the thumb and fingers.

Q 4. To which varieties of synovial joints do these joints belong and what movements occur at them? *2 marks*

Joint	Variety of synovial joint	Movement
Interphalangeal joint of thumb	Hinge (½ mark)	Flexion/extension (½ mark)
Metacarpophalangeal joint of finger	Ellipsoidal joint (½ mark)	Flexion/extension + abduction/ adduction (½ mark)

Q 5. Only one muscle of the forearm attaches to a carpal bone. Which muscle is this and to which bone does it directly attach? *2 marks*

A Flexor carpi ulnaris (1 mark). It attaches to the pisiform (1 mark).

Q 6. Explain how a fracture heals. *6 marks*

A Any 12 of the following points (awarded ½ mark each):

1. Formation of fracture haematoma (½ mark) with necrosis of bone immediately adjacent to fracture (½ mark). Fibroblasts infiltrate the blood clot (organisation) (½ mark).

2. Subperiosteal and endosteal cellular proliferation (½ mark) with cellular tissue forming from each side of the fracture (½ mark). The blood clot is absorbed and takes little or no part in the repair process (½ mark).

3. Callus formation (½ mark) when osteoprogenitor cells are stimulated to proliferate (½ mark) and become osteoblasts (½ mark), which lay down osteoid (½ mark) that is calcified (½ mark) to become woven bone (callus) (½ mark).

4. Consolidation (½ mark) when osteoblasts continue the repair process, replacing woven bone with lamellar bone (½ mark).

5. Remodelling (½ mark). Bone is resorbed (½ mark) and lamellar bone is deposited (½ mark) thus restoring bone to near normal form (½ mark). Osteoclasts are important in remodelling (½ mark).

Q 7. In the radiograph above (Figure 5.3), what are the radiolucent lines across the distal ends of the radius and the ulna and at the proximal end of the first metacarpal? *1 mark*

A Epiphyseal (growth) plates.

Q 8. Why are such regions not visible in the second to fifth metacarpals in the above radiograph? *1 mark*

A Because they occur at the heads of the bones that are outside the field of the radiographs.

Q 9. Chondrocytes are found in these radiolucent regions. What changes do these cells undergo at these sites? *4 marks*

A They proliferate (1 mark), arrange themselves in columns (1 mark), hypertrophy (enlarge) (1 mark) and degenerate (apoptosis) (1 mark).

Q 10. Define the terms 'diaphysis' and 'metaphysis'. *2 marks*

A Diaphysis: the shaft of a long bone (1 mark) or the part of a long bone formed from the primary centre of ossification (1 mark).

A Metaphysis: the region of most recently laid down bone (1 mark) or the part of the diaphysis adjacent to the epiphyseal plate (1 mark).

Q 11. The ossification centres of the hand are useful in forensic work for establishing the age of juvenile subjects. What stage of formation have the carpal bones reached at the time of birth?   *1 mark*

A Usually, all the carpal bones are still at the stage of cartilage models at birth.

Following fracture at the waist of the scaphoid bone, part of the scaphoid bone may undergo avascular necrosis.

Q 12. Which part of the scaphoid bone is usually affected by avascular necrosis and why?   *2 marks*

A The proximal part (1 mark). The blood vessels of the scaphoid bone enter the more distal part and run proximally (1 mark).

📖 REFERENCES

Crawford Adams J. Hamblen D L. 1999. *Outline of Fractures*, 11th edn. Edinburgh: Churchill Livingstone.

Scheuer L, Black S. 2000. *Developmental Juvenile Osteology*. London: Elsevier Academic Press.

Scothorne R J. 1976. Early development. In Passmore R, Robson J S (eds). *A Companion to Medical Studies,* 2nd edn., Vol. 1, chapter 19. Oxford: Blackwell Scientific Publications.

Solomon L, Warwick D, Nayagam S. 2001. *Apley's System of Orthopaedics and Fractures*, 8th edn. London: Arnold.

MUSCULOSKELETAL
3. SPINE

Mr Martin, a 30-year-old teacher, has presented with low back pain of sudden onset. Over the school holidays he has been building a garden wall. The back pain came on when he attempted to lift a bag of cement. There was also a sensation of 'something giving'. The pain is in his lower back and is radiating to the perineum and down the backs of both thighs towards his calves. Mr Martin complains that the pain in his legs feels worse than that in his back. There is also a sensation of tingling down the back of the thigh and he has noticed that he has become numb at the lower part of his buttocks and around the region of his genitalia and anus. He has become incontinent of faeces and has not passed urine in the two hours since the injury.

Q **1. What is the most likely diagnosis for Mr Martin?** *2 mark*

A Central (1 mark) prolapse (1 mark) of an intervertebral disc.

On examination, sensory loss is detected on the back of both thighs and across the perineum. Motor function of both his lower limbs is difficult to assess because of the pain, but Mr Martin seems to be having particular difficulty moving his ankles. Ankle jerk reflexes are diminished, although knee jerk reflexes seem normal. An attempt to lift each leg passively from the bed with Mr Martin supine, the straight leg raise test, is also painful. It is also noted that Mr Martin has a palpable urinary bladder but is unable to pass urine (urinary retention) for which a catheter is passed.

Q **2. Which spinal nerves are involved in the knee-jerk and ankle-jerk reflexes?** *1 marks*

A Knee-jerk: L2, L3 (½ mark). Ankle jerk: S1, S2 (½ mark).

MUSCULOSKELETAL

Q 3. Why did the straight leg raise test elicit pain? *1 mark*

A It puts tension on the sciatic nerve and thus irritates the affected spinal nerve(s).

Q 4. On the basis of motor signs, which nerve roots are most likely to have been affected by the prolapsed disc? Give reasons for your answer. *3 marks*

A The sacral (½ mark) spinal nerve roots in general (½ mark) seem to have been affected. These roots are important in supplying the muscles that flex (½ mark) and extend (½ mark) the ankle and these muscles seem weak. The ankle jerk reflexes on both sides are weak (½ mark). The ano-rectal and bladder dysfunction (½ mark) also suggest involvement of sacral nerves as these organs are also supplied by the sacral spinal nerves.

Q 5. Involvement of which spinal nerves is suggested by the sensory loss? Give reasons for your answer. *2 marks*

A The numbness on the back of the thigh (½ mark) and perineum (½ mark) is consistent with dysfunction of S2 (½ mark) to S4 (½ mark) spinal nerves.

Q 6. Are the root values suggested by the motor and sensory signs consistent with the positive straight leg raise test? *1 mark*

A Yes. The straight leg raise irritates the sciatic nerve which has root values L4, L5, S1, S2, S3.

Q 7. Which component of the intervertebral disc is it that prolapses? *1 mark*

A The nucleus pulposus (1 mark) prolapses through the annulus fibrosus.

Q 8. Identify features A–F on the following diagram (Figure 5.4). *3 marks*

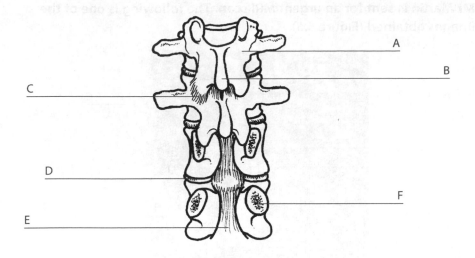

Figure 5.4: Anatomy of the spine.

A ½ mark for each:

A – Lamina

B – Spinous process

C – Facet joint

D – Intervertebral disc

E – Posterior longitudinal ligament

F – Pedicle

In Mr Martin the disc has prolapsed centrally. It is more common (and less serious) for the disc to prolapse posterolaterally rather than passing directly posteriorly in the midline as in Mr Martin.

Q 9. Why does a disc tend to prolapse posterolaterally? *2 marks*

A The posterior longitudinal ligament (1 mark) attaches firmly to the posterior aspect of the intervertebral disc (1 mark) so that the prolapse is forced to occur to one side of the midline.

Mr Martin is sent for an urgent MRI scan. The following is one of the images obtained (Figure 5.5).

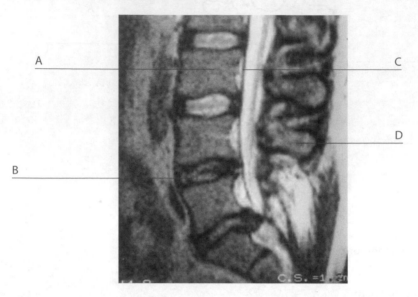

Figure 5.5: Mr Martin's MRI scan.

Q 10. On the image, identify A–D.   *4 marks*

A 1 mark for each:

A – Vertebral body (½ mark) of L3 (½ mark)

B – L4/L5 intervertebral disc

C – Posterior longitudinal ligament

D – Spinous process of L4

Q 11. Which disc has prolapsed?   *1 mark*

A L5/S1 disc.

Q 12. Which component of the nervous system is found in the vertebral canal at this level? *1 mark*

A The cauda equina.

📁 **LEARNING POINT**

The spinal cord terminates at the level of the L1/L2 intervertebral disc. The cauda equina consists of the dorsal and ventral roots of the lower spinal nerves as they pass inferiorly to exit from the vertebral canal.

Q 13. Where does the L4 spinal nerve exit from the vertebral canal? *1 mark*

A At the intervertebral foramen between the pedicles of L4 and L5 vertebrae.

Q 14. How does S1 spinal nerve exit from the vertebral canal? *2 marks*

A The dorsal and ventral roots of S1 unite within the sacral canal to form the spinal nerve proper. It soon divides into its dorsal and ventral rami (1 mark) which exit from the canal through the dorsal and ventral sacral foramina (1 mark).

Q 15. What is the lowest limit of the cerebrospinal fluid in the vertebral canal? *1 mark*

A CSF is found as far down as S2 vertebra (1 mark) where the dural sac, and thus the lumbar cistern of CSF, terminates.

Q 16. Which nerves are responsible for maintenance of anal tone and what are their root values? *2 marks*

A The left and right pudendal nerves (1 mark) supply the skeletal muscle of the anal sphincter. The root values of the pudendal nerve is S2, S3 and S4 (1 mark).

MUSCULOSKELETAL

Q 17. Which nerves supply the detrusor muscle of the bladder? From which spinal nerves do they arise?   *2 marks*

A The smooth muscle of the bladder is supplied by the pelvic splanchnic (parasympathetic) nerves (1 mark). They arise from S2, S3 and S4 spinal nerves (1 mark).

As a result of central prolapse pressing on the cauda equina, Mr Martin is diagnosed as having cauda equina syndrome and is referred for urgent neurosurgical decompression.

📖 BIBLIOGRAPHY

Crawford Adams J. Hamblen D L. 2001. *Outline of Orthopaedics*, 13th edn. Edinburgh: Churchill Livingstone.

Ellis H. 2002. *Clinical Anatomy*, 10th edn. Oxford: Blackwell Publishing.

Solomon L, Warwick D, Nayagam S. 2001. *Apley's System of Orthopaedics and Fractures*, 8th edn. London: Arnold.

Standring S. 2005. *Gray's Anatomy*, 39th edn. Edinburgh: Elsevier Churchill Livingstone.

MUSCULOSKELETAL

MUSCULOSKELETAL
4. HERNIA

You are a surgical house officer and you are clerking in Mr Henderson who is being admitted for an elective open hernia repair.

While you are taking a history from Mr Henderson, he asks you what a hernia is.

Q 1. What is a hernia? *1 mark*

A A hernia occurs when part or all of a structure protrudes through the tissue in which it is normally contained.

Mr Henderson tells you that he was quite alarmed when he found a lump in his groin and was rather relieved when his GP told him it was a hernia and not something more serious.

Q 2. What is the differential diagnosis of a groin lump? *3 marks*

A ½ mark for each of the following:

Inguinal hernia

Femoral hernia

Lymphadenopathy

Femoral aneurysm

Undescended testicle

Saphena varix

Lipoma

Q 3. On your examination, how would you distinguish an inguinal hernia from a femoral hernia? *2 marks*

A Inguinal hernia: The neck of an inguinal hernia lies above and medial to the pubic tubercle, above the inguinal ligament.

A Femoral hernia: The hernia lies below and lateral to the pubic tubercle, below the inguinal ligament.

You make a note that Mr Henderson has a right inguinal hernia. You also document that the hernia is 'reducible'.

Q 4. What does this term mean? *1 mark*

A This means the contents of the hernia can be returned to the abdominal cavity when the patient lies down or when you apply pressure over it.

📂 LEARNING POINT

If a hernia is irreducible, it cannot be returned into the abdominal cavity. This occurs when the contents of the hernial sac become swollen due to the constriction of the neck of the hernia as it passes through the abdominal wall.

Q 5. List three complications of an irreducible hernia. Explain how they occur. *6 marks*

Complication	Marks	Explanation	Marks
Obstruction	1	The hernia contains a loop of bowel that becomes oedematous and leads to bowel obstruction	1
Strangulation	1	The blood supply of the piece of bowel is compromised	1
Peritonitis	1	Due to sepsis spreading from the compromised bowel	1

You wonder if it is a **direct** or an **indirect** inguinal hernia.

Q 6. How would you distinguish between these on clinical examination?

3 marks

A Reduce the hernia, if possible, and press over the deep ring (1 mark). Ask the patient to cough (1 mark). A protrusion medial to the deep inguinal ring suggests a direct hernia (1 mark).

 LEARNING POINT

An indirect hernia passes through the deep inguinal ring so it will not protrude on coughing when pressure is exerted on the abdominal wall at the deep ring. A direct inguinal hernia bulges forward directly through the posterior wall of the inguinal canal medial to the deep ring. Sometimes it can be difficult to distinguish between a direct and an indirect inguinal hernia on clinical examination.

Indirect inguinal hernia

This can be a congenital hernia due to a patent processus vaginalis (the peritoneal sac which migrates along with the testis as it enters the scrotum in late fetal life). It may also be due to a hernial sac forming in later life.

Direct inguinal hernia

Found mainly in the older age group due to abdominal wall weakness at the conjoint tendon. Is often bilateral. Not as prone to complications as an indirect inguinal hernia.

Femoral hernia

More common in females. Often strangulates.

You are keen to pursue a career in surgery and manage to get time from your ward duties to observe Mr Henderson's operation in theatre. Your consultant, tells you that the femoral artery can be used as a landmark to determine the position of the deep ring.

Q 7. Where can the femoral artery be palpated? Give your answer in relation to bony landmarks.   *1 mark*

A The femoral artery is palpable mid-way between the anterior superior iliac spine and pubic symphysis (1 mark). This is called the mid-inguinal point.

Q 8. If inserting a needle into the femoral artery to collect arterial blood, it is important to appreciate the relationship of the femoral artery to the femoral nerve and femoral vein. What is this relationship?   *1 mark*

A The femoral nerve lies lateral to the artery and the vein lies medial to the artery.

📁 LEARNING POINT

Remembering the relationship between the femoral nerve, artery and vein can be assisted by two mnemonics:

VAN: vein – artery – nerve from medial to lateral

or

NAVY: nerve – artery – vein – Y-fronts(!) from lateral to medial

---

Q 9. What is the position of the deep inguinal ring? Give your answer in relation to bony landmarks.   *1 mark*

A The deep inguinal ring lies above the inguinal ligament mid-way between the anterior superior iliac spine and the pubic tubercle.

Q 10. What is the position of the deep ring in relation to the femoral artery?   *1 mark*

A The deep ring lies immediately lateral to and 2 cm superior to the femoral artery.

Q 11. In this patient what structure passes through the deep inguinal ring that allows it to be easily identified by the surgeon? *1 mark*

A The spermatic cord.

The consultant continues to quiz your anatomical knowledge by asking you about the important structures in the inguinal canal.

Q 12. Name two structures in this patient's inguinal canal that a surgeon would take particular care to avoid damaging. *1 mark*

A Ilioinguinal nerve (½ mark)

A Spermatic cord (½ mark)

Q 13. Name four structures that lie within the spermatic cord. *2 marks*

A ½ mark for any four of the following:

Ductus deferens

Testicular artery

Pampiniform plexus of testicular veins

Epididymal vessels

Lymphatic vessels

Autonomic nerves

Q 14. Please identify structures A–H on this diagram (Figure 5.6) of the inguinal canal. *4 marks*

MUSCULOSKELETAL

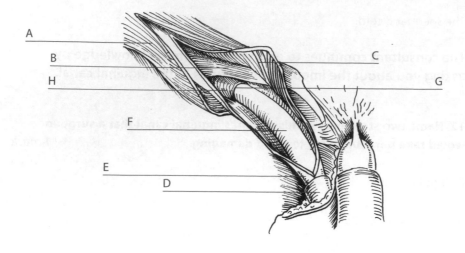

A

B

H

C

G

F

E

D

MUSCULOSKELETAL

Figure 5.6: The inguinal canal.

A ½ mark for each of the following:

A – External oblique aponeurosis

B – Transversus abdominis muscle

C – Internal oblique muscle

D – External spermatic fascia

E – Cremasteric fascia

F – Spermatic cord

G –Deep inguinal ring

H – Tranversalis fascia

Q **15. The hernial sac is found to lie medial to the inferior epigastric vessels. Is the hernia direct or indirect?** *1 mark*

A Direct (1 mark) because the sac has passed directly through the posterior wall of the inguinal canal, the region medial to the inferior epigastric vessels.

The surgeon repairs the hernia by strengthening the conjoint tendon.

Q **16. What is the conjoint tendon and where does it lie in relation to the inguinal canal?** *1 mark*

A The conjoint tendon (inguinal falx) is the common aponeurosis of the tranversus abdominis and internal oblique muscles (½ mark). It lies in the posterior wall of the inguinal canal (½ mark).

📖 BIBLIOGRAPHY

Ellis H. 2002. *Clinical Anatomy*, 10th edn. Oxford: Blackwell Publishing.

Last R J, Sinnatamby C S. 1999. *Last's Anatomy: Regional and Applied*, 10th edn. Edinburgh: Churchill Livingstone.

Monkhouse S. 2001. *Clinical Anatomy*. Edinburgh: Churchill Livingstone.

MUSCULOSKELETAL
5. HIP FRACTURE

You are the Foundation Year 2 receiving doctor on the orthopaedic ward in a busy general hospital when Mrs Smith, a 76-year-old woman, is referred to you from the Accident and Emergency Department. Earlier in the day she had tripped on an uneven pavement and fallen on to her left side. She is now complaining of pain in her groin and thigh. The pain radiates to the knee. Mrs Smith is unable to weight-bear.

Q **1. From the history, what is the most likely diagnosis for Mrs Smith and explain your reasoning.** *2 marks*

A The most likely diagnosis is fractured neck of femur (1 mark).

A ½ mark for any two of the following:

A Elderly woman or woman with osteoporosis (½ mark); had a fall (½ mark); cannot weight-bear (½ mark); pain in groin and thigh (½ mark).

An X-ray was taken (Figure 5.7) and the diagnosis confirmed.

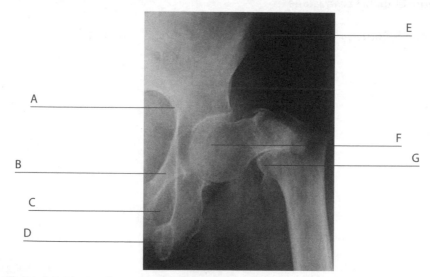

Figure 5.7: Mrs Smith's X-ray.

Q 2. *7 marks*

A – Pelvic brim

B – Superior ramus of pubis

C – Obturator foramen

D – Ischial tuberosity

E – Anterior superior iliac spine

F – Head of femur

G – Lesser trochanter

The hip joint is innervated by branches of the femoral nerve, obturator nerve, accessory obturator nerve when present, and of the nerve to quadratus femoris. This helps explain the distribution of the pain.

Q 3. Why, as in Mrs Smith, does pain from the hip sometimes radiate to the knee? *1 mark*

A The hip and knee joints both (½ mark) receive innervation from the femoral and obturator nerves (½ mark).

☞ LEARNING POINT

This is an example of referred pain. The femoral and obturator nerves arise from the ventral rami of L2, L3 and L4 spinal nerves. In some patients pain from hip disease is only felt in the knee!!

Q 4. What is Hilton's Law[a]? *2 marks*

A Hilton's Law states that, in general, the nerve supplying a joint also supplies the muscles that move the joint (1 mark) and the skin (1 mark) covering the articular insertion of those muscles.

After a diagnosis has been established you start to consider whether there may be associated complications.

Q **5. List two acute complications that may follow fractured neck of femur.** *2 marks*

A Any two of the following:

Fat embolism (1 mark)

Avascular necrosis (1 mark)

Hypovolaemic shock (1 mark) – massive bleeding

Q **6. What is the main source of arterial blood supply of the head of the femur?** *1 mark*

A The trochanteric anastomosis.

 LEARNING POINT

The trochanteric anastomosis lies close to the greater trochanter. It receives blood from the superior and (usually) the inferior gluteal arteries and ascending branches of the medial and lateral circumflex femoral arteries. Blood will also pass through vessels within the bone and there is a very small contribution from the ligament of the head of the femur.

Q **7. What are the retinacular fibres of the hip joint capsule?** *1 mark*

A The retinacular fibres are fibres that are reflected from the femoral part of the capsular attachment up the neck of the femur (1 mark) within the capsule.

Q **8. What is their relationship to the blood supply of the head of the femur?** *1 mark*

A The blood vessels of the head of the femur lie deep to them.

MUSCULOSKELETAL

On further examination of Mrs Smith you find her left leg to be shortened and laterally (externally) rotated. This is due to muscle contraction.

Q 9. Name a muscle that laterally rotates the hip.   *1 mark*

A Obturator externus and internus, the gemelli and quadratus femoris, piriformis, gluteus maximus and sartorius (1 mark for any one).

 LEARNING POINT

It is hard to know precisely which muscle(s) is(are) responsible for the lateral rotation of the hip seen in Mrs Smith. Lateral rotation tends to be more powerful than medial rotation. Several muscles work together to produce this movement. Following a fracture the bones may be displaced so that the muscle pull is altered.

Mrs Smith had her hip surgically repaired by a hemiarthroplasty and began a programme of early mobilisation while recovering in hospital.

Q 10. What is a hemiarthroplasty?   *1 mark*

A Only one-half of the joint is replaced (1 mark) by a prosthetic joint surface.

For one of the exercises, the physiotherapist told Mrs Smith to lie on her back, slide her foot up towards her buttock, bending her hip and knee (Figure 5.8).

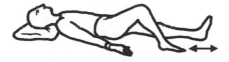

Figure 5.8: Physiotherapy exercises after hemiarthroplasty.

Q **11. Which muscle is the principal flexor of the hip?** *1 mark*

A Psoas major (1 mark) or iliopsoas (1 mark).

Q **12. Which three individual muscles are the principal flexors of the knee?** *1½ marks*

A Biceps femoris (½ mark), semitendinosus (½ mark) and semimembranosus (1 mark) (hamstrings) are the principal flexors of the knee, although others assist in the movement.

Before Mrs Smith is discharged from hospital, she undergoes a dual-energy X-ray absorptiometry (DEXA) scan. It confirms that she is suffering from osteoporosis.

Q **13. Which cells of bone lay down new bone?** *½ mark*

A Osteoblasts.

Q **14. The table below indicates a number of features of osteocytes, osteoblasts and osteoclasts. In the right-hand column indicate of which cell type each of the features is characteristic.** *4 marks*

A ½ mark for each

Feature	Bone cell
Abundant lysosomes	Osteoclast
Abundant rough endoplasmic reticulum	Osteoblast
Basophilic cytoplasm	Osteoblast
Cellular processes in canaliculi	Osteocyte
Howship's lacuna	Osteoclast
Lie between bony lamellae	Osteocyte
Multiple nuclei	Osteoclast
Ruffled border	Osteoclast

MUSCULOSKELETAL

LEARNING POINT

Cells producing protein, such as the collagen-producing osteoblasts, are rich in ribosomes. In cells where the protein is to be secreted from the cell, the ribosomes are on the rough endoplasmic reticulum. The ribosomes are composed of ribonucleic acid and thus stain heavily with alkaline dyes, giving basophilic cytoplasm on histology.

Review of Mrs Smith's most recent post-operative blood results showed a profile compatible with a diagnosis of osteoporosis.

Q 15. Which of the following sets of results are Mrs Smith's? Explain your answer. *2 marks*

	A	B	C	Normal range
Ca	2.3 mmol/l	2.5 mmol/l	1.9 mmol/l	2.20–2.67 mmol/l
PO$_4$	1.1 mmol/l	1.2 mmol/l	0.7 mmol/l	0.8–1.5 mmol/l
Alk. Phos.	1070 IU/ml	80 IU/l	205 IU/l	39–117 IU/l

A The correct answer is B (1 mark).

A Osteoporosis is a reduction of bone density. It is of such slow progression that no biochemical abnormalities are detectable in the blood (1 mark).

LEARNING POINT

A – Paget's disease[b]

B – Mrs Smith

C – Osteomalacia

Mrs Smith is prescribed calcium supplements and a bisphosphonate for her osteoporosis.

MUSCULOSKELETAL

Q 16. How do bisphosphonates work?   *2 marks*

A Any of the following up to 2 marks:

Decreases the rate of bone turnover (1 mark).

Inhibits recruitment (½ mark) and function of osteoclasts (½ mark).

Promotes apoptosis of osteoclasts (½ mark).

📖 BIBLIOGRAPHY

Crawford Adams J. Hamblen D L. 1999. *Outline of Fractures*, 11th edn. Edinburgh: Churchill Livingstone.

Ellis H. 2002. *Clinical Anatomy*, 10th edn. Oxford: Blackwell Publishing.

Kumar P, Clark M. 2005. *Clinical Medicine*, 6th edn. Edinburgh: Elsevier Saunders.

Last R J, Sinnatamby C S. 1999. *Last's Anatomy: Regional and Applied*, 10th edn. Edinburgh: Churchill Livingstone.

Provan D, Krentz A. 2002. *Oxford Handbook of Clinical and Laboratory Investigation*. Oxford: Oxford University Press.

[a]John Hilton (1805–1934), surgeon at Guy's Hospital London, described the innervation of joints. He was President of the Royal College of Surgeons of England in 1867 and surgeon extraordinary to Queen Victoria.

[b]James Paget (1814–1899), British pathologist, remembered for Paget's disease of bone and Paget's disease of the nipple. Like Hilton, Paget was President of the Royal College of Surgeons of England in 1875 and surgeon extraordinary to Queen Victoria.

MUSCULOSKELETAL

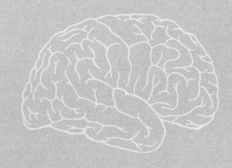

NEUROLOGY CASES:
ANSWERS

NEUROLOGY
1. MOTOR NEURON DISEASE

You are on duty at a local hospice. 34-year-old Mr Wilson, is admitted for one week of respite care. It is your duty to clerk him in. Mr Wilson was diagnosed with motor neuron disease 18 months ago.

Q 1. What is motor neuron disease? *½ mark*

A Motor neuron disease is a degenerative neurological disease.

Q 2. Which components of the central nervous system (CNS) are affected in motor neuron disease? *1½ marks*

A Neurons in the motor cortex (½ mark), cranial nerve nuclei (½ mark) and anterior horn cells/corticospinal tracts (½ mark) within the spinal cord.

📁 LEARNING POINT

The cause of motor neuron disease is unknown. Oxidative damage, abnormal protein aggregation and abnormal axonal transport are all thought to be involved. The incidence is around 2/100 000 per annum and it is slightly more common in males. The typical age of onset is 30–40 years. There is no cure for motor neuron disease and the patient's condition deteriorates progressively. Survival from diagnosis is rarely more than three years.

Q 3. In which pathways from the motor cortex do most motor impulses descend? *1 mark*

A Lateral and anterior corticospinal tracts (½ mark) and the corticonuclear (corticobulbar) tracts (½ mark).

NEUROLOGY

LEARNING POINT

A small amount of motor activity may be mediated by the vestibulospinal, rubrospinal and tectospinal tracts.

Q 4. What is a motor unit?   *1 mark*

A A single somatic (lower) motor neuron (½ mark) and all the muscle fibres it stimulates (½ mark).

Since motor neuron disease affects motor neurons, the clinical manifestations are primarily within skeletal muscles rather than in smooth or cardiac muscle.

Q 5. Complete the following table comparing the three muscle types. *6 marks*

	Skeletal	Cardiac	Smooth
Striated or non-striated?	Striated (½ mark)	Striated (½ mark)	Non-striated (½ mark)
Peripheral or central nucleus/nuclei?	Peripheral (½ mark)	Central (½ mark)	Central (½ mark)
Single or multiple nuclei?	Multiple (½ mark)	Single (½ mark)	Single (½ mark)
Small, large or very large fibre diameter?	Very large (½ mark)	Large (½ mark)	Small (½ mark)

After taking a full and detailed history, you examine Mr Wilson. During the examination of the nervous system, you find that in Mr Wilson's upper limbs there are muscle wasting, fasciculation and reduced power in all muscle groups.

Q 6. What do the fasciculations indicate?   *1 mark*

A That lower motor neurons have been affected.

NEUROLOGY

LEARNING POINT

Fasciculations are small involuntary contractions of a motor unit. They are a feature of lower motor neuron disease. They can only be seen if the muscle is relaxed.

You continue with the neurological examination and find there is also reduced power in the lower limbs.

Q 7. Label the following diagram (Figure 6.1) of the calf muscles of the right lower limb.   *3 marks*

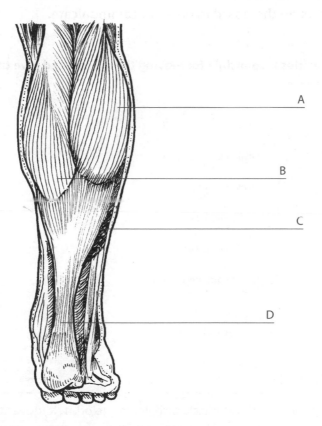

Figure 6.1: Anatomy of the calf muscles of the right lower limb.

A – Lateral head of the gastrocnemius (½ mark).

B – Medial head of the gastrocnemius (½ mark).

C – Soleus (1 mark).

D – Calcaneal/Achilles tendon (1 mark).

After examining Mr Wilson you present your findings to the on-call consultant. You note that there was no involvement of the extraocular muscles. The consultant explains to you that in motor neuron disease the extraocular muscles are often not involved and, if they are, it is a very late feature of the disease. She also tells you that in patients with advanced motor neuron disease, movement of the eyeball is often the only means of communication. Special boards are used which allow the patient to spell out words by looking at letters on the board in order to communicate.

Q **8. List the six muscles responsible for moving the eyeball and give the nerve supply of each.** *3 marks*

Superior rectus	Oculomotor nerve/CN III
Inferior rectus	Oculomotor nerve/CN III
Medial rectus	Oculomotor nerve/CN III
Lateral rectus	Abducens nerve/CN VI
Superior oblique	Trochlear nerve/CN IV
Inferior oblique	Oculomotor nerve/CN III

A ½ mark for each muscle and its innervation.

📁 **LEARNING POINT**

The levator palpebrae superioris muscle also lies in the orbit. It moves the eyelids rather than the eyeball and is supplied by the oculomotor nerve.

NEUROLOGY

Mr Wilson's wife explains that a few months ago he lost the ability to chew and swallow safely. He had lost almost a stone in weight before a percutaneous endoscopic gastrostomy (PEG) tube was inserted by the surgical team.

Q 9. What is a PEG tube? *1 mark*

A A PEG tube allows a nutrient solution to be passed directly into the stomach (1 mark) alleviating the need to chew or swallow food.

Q 10. Label the muscles that are shown in this illustration (Figure 6.2). *2 marks*

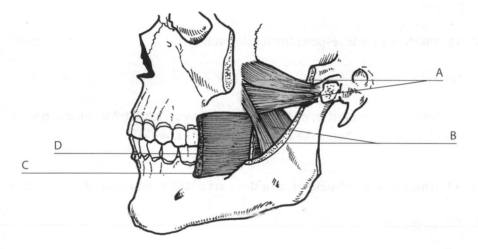

Figure 6.2: Some muscles of chewing and swallowing

A ½ mark for each of the following:

A – Lateral pterygoid.

B – Medial pterygoid.

C – Buccinator.

D – Superior constrictor.

Q 11. What is the innervation of the 'muscles of mastication'?   *1 mark*

A Mandibular nerve/trigeminal nerve/CN V.

During examination of Mr Wilson's cranial nerves, you find abnormalities of the facial nerve. You find he can only raise his eyebrows minimally and not against resistance.

Q 12. Which muscle is responsible for raising the eyebrows?   *1 mark*

A Frontalis/occipto-frontalis muscle.

You notice that Mr Wilson is also unable to close his eyes tightly.

Q 13. Which muscle is responsible for this action?   *1 mark*

A Orbicularis oculi.

On further examination of the facial nerve you notice Mr Wilson has great difficulty when asked to 'blow out his cheeks'.

Q 14. Which muscle is being used in this part of the examination?   *1 mark*

A Orbicularis oris.

 LEARNING POINT

A common misconception is that asking a patient to 'blow out his/her cheeks' is testing the buccinator muscles. The test actually relies upon pursing of the lips to create an airtight seal, which involves the orbicularis oris.

As well as supplying the muscles of facial expression, the facial nerve has sensory and autonomic functions.

Q 15. What are the sensory and autonomic functions of the facial nerve? *2 marks*

A Sensory – taste (½ mark) from the anterior two-thirds of the tongue (½ mark).

A Autonomic – the secretion of saliva (½ mark) and tears (½ mark).

🗁 LEARNING POINT

Parasympathetic fibres in the facial nerve stimulate the secretion of saliva from only the submandibular, sublingual and minor glands. The parotid gland is innervated by parasympathetic fibres in the glossopharyngeal nerve.

Nearing completion of your examination of the cranial nerves you find that Mr Wilson is unable to shrug his shoulders.

Q 16. Which cranial nerves are responsible for this action? *1 mark*

A The spinal accessory nerves

Q 17. The following diagram (Figure 6.3) shows the attachments of the cranial nerves to the brain. Identify structures A–F. *3 marks*

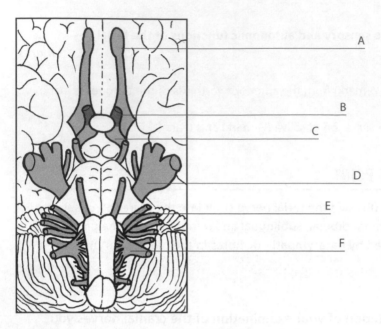

Figure 6.3: Attachments of the cranial nerves to the brain.

A ½ mark for each of the following:

A – Olfactory bulb.

B – Optic nerve.

C – Optic tract.

D – Trigeminal nerve.

E – Abducens nerve.

F – Hypoglossal nerve.

📖 BIBLIOGRAPHY

Hiatt J L, Gartner L P. 2000. *Textbook of Head and Neck Anatomy*, 3rd edn. New York: Lippincott, Williams and Wilkins.

Johnson D R, Moore W J. 1997. *Anatomy for Dental Students*, 3rd edn. Oxford: Oxford University Press.

Kiernan J A. 2005. *Barr's The Human Nervous System: An Anatomical Viewpoint*, 8th edn. Philadelphia: Lippincott Williams and Wilkins.

Standring S. 2005. *Gray's Anatomy*, 39th edn. Edinburgh: Elsevier Churchill Livingstone.

Tortora G J, Grabowski S. 2002. *Principles of Anatomy and Physiology*, 10th edn. New York: John Wiley.

NEUROLOGY
2. CEREBRAL ARTERY DISEASE

You are working in general practice when 61-year-old Mr Johnston comes to see you complaining of having 'funny turns' recently. He describes two episodes which occurred within the last three weeks. He explains that during the first episode the vision in his left eye became 'foggy' for about two minutes. During the next episode his vision 'went funny' again and he became weak down his right side. This also lasted a few minutes. Following both episodes Mr Johnston was well. Further questioning reveals that the weakness particularly affected his right hand and right lower limb. The visual disturbance in the second attack was not the same as in the first. The first time only Mr Johnston's left eye was affected and the sight was completely lost for the duration of the attack. The second time the attack affected both eyes and he seemed to lose the right side of his field of vision in both eyes.

Q 1. What is the most likely diagnosis of the first episode when Mr Johnston had visual impairment in his left eye?   *1 mark*

A Amaurosis fugax.

Q 2. What is the most likely diagnosis of the second episode?   *1 mark*

A Transient ischaemic attack.

Q 3. Where are the sites of ischaemia likely to be in the first and second episodes? Explain your reasoning.   *4 marks*

A In the first episode only the left eye is affected suggesting ischaemia of the left retina or optic nerve (1 mark). In the second episode loss of the right side of the field of vision is accompanied by right-sided weakness of both the upper and lower limbs. The combination indicates ischaemia in the cerebral hemisphere (1 mark). The visual and motor pathways are both crossed (1 mark), ie visual information from the right side passes to the left hemisphere and the right upper and lower limbs are controlled from the left hemisphere. The ischaemia must thus be in the left (1 mark) cerebral hemisphere. The motor and visual pathways run close together in the region of the internal capsule (1 mark) and thus this is the most likely site. (Students need to get 4 out of the 5 options for full marks.)

 LEARNING POINT

Amaurosis fugax refers to a transient loss of vision in one eye. It is a common, painless symptom and implies transient retinal ischaemia. It is usually associated with emboli or stenosis of the ipsilateral internal carotid artery.

A transient ischaemic attack is an episode where there is a temporary loss of brain function due to vascular insufficiency. Most transient ischaemic attacks last about 30 min, with a complete recovery within 24 hours.

Symptoms from a transient ischaemic attack originating in the anterior (internal carotid) circulation include dysphasia, one-sided motor weakness in the upper and/or lower limb, a hemisensory deficit and visual disturbance. Transient symptoms originating from the posterior (vertebral artery) circulation include ataxia, amnesia, vertigo and diplopia.

On examination, you find Mr Johnston to be well. He is a heavy man with central obesity and a ruddy complexion. His pulse is regular with a rate of 82 beats per minute and his blood pressure is 172/94 mmHg. You also notice that Mr Johnston has xanthelasma and corneal arcus, but there are no further cardiovascular findings to note. Neurological examination is normal.

Q 4. What is xanthelasma and what is its clinical significance?   *1 mark*

A Xanthelasma is an adipose deposit at the eyelids (½ mark). It is associated with hyperlipidaemia or hypercholesterolaemia (½ mark).

NEUROLOGY

Q **5. Is the corneal arcus (arcus senilis) significant?** *1 mark*

A Not really. It is very common in older people (1 mark) but would warrant investigation in younger patients.

You start Mr Johnson on aspirin and after an ECG, repeat blood pressure measurements and carry out further assessment of his blood cholesterol/lipoprotein levels. You also prescribe a statin for his cholesterol and a thiazide diuretic for his blood pressure.

Q **6. Describe how these drugs work.** *3 marks*

A 1 mark per drug

Drug	Mechanism of action
Aspirin	Aspirin is an antiplatelet drug (½ mark). It inhibits thromboxane A2 in platelets (½ mark), and prostacyclin in endothelial walls (½ mark)
Statin	Statins are lipid-modulating drugs (½ mark) that inhibit the enzyme HMG CoA reductase (½ mark) involved in cholesterol biosynthesis (½ mark). This results in decreased plasma cholesterol and increased LDL receptors (½ mark)
Thiazide diuretic	Thiazide diuretics inhibit sodium reabsorption (½ mark) in the proximal convoluted tubule (½ mark), reducing water reabsorption and thus blood pressure (½ mark)

Mr Johnston also has carotid Doppler[a] ultrasound studies which show stenosis at the lower end of the left internal carotid.

Q **7. What arteries arise from the internal carotid artery in the cranial cavity?** *4 marks*

A Ophthalmic artery (1 mark), anterior cerebral artery (1 mark), middle cerebral artery (1 mark) and posterior communicating artery (1 mark).

NEUROLOGY

Q 8. On the following diagram (Figure 6.4) indicate the location of: the central sulcus, the lateral fissure and the primary motor cortex. Indicate the regions of the motor cortex that serve (A) the upper limb, (B) the lower limb and (C) the head and neck. *6 marks*

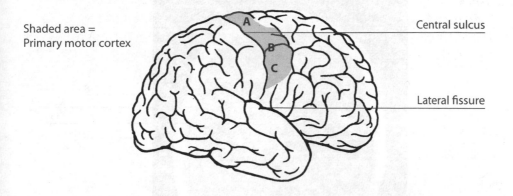

Shaded area =
Primary motor cortex

Central sulcus

Lateral fissure

Figure 6.4: Surface anatomy of the brain.

A – Lower limb area.

B – Upper limb area.

C – Head and neck area.

Q 9. In neuroanatomy, what is meant by the term somatotopic localisation? *1 mark*

A Somatotopic localisation is the concept that certain regions of the nervous system mediate neurological function in certain parts of the body.

Mr Johnston is referred to the vascular surgeons.

You recall seeing a patient when you worked in hospital where undetected embolic disease resulted in a stroke. The 70-year-old patient presented with a left hemiplegia. One of the CT scan views is shown below (Figure 6.5).

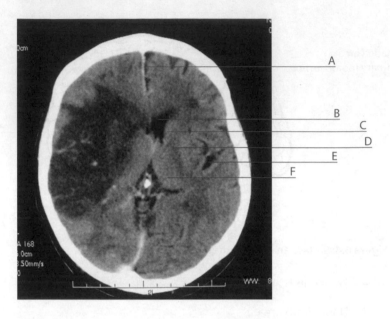

Figure 6.5: CT scan.

Q 10. On the CT scan identify A–F.   *6 marks*

A – Falx cerebri.

B – Lateral ventricle.

C – Caudate nucleus.

D – Internal capsule.

E – Lateral fissure.

F – Thalamus.

Q 11. Why did this patient have a left hemiplegia?   *2 marks*

A Because the infarction affected the right (1 mark) internal capsule (1 mark).

LEARNING POINT

Cerebrovascular accidents lead to infarction and loss of function of the brain region supplied by particular blood vessels. In understanding the site of a brain lesion it is important to appreciate that loss of motor function could result from loss of motor cortex through occlusion of the anterior (lower limb region of motor cortex) or middle (upper limb/head and neck region of motor cortex) cerebral arteries or through damage to the more inferiorly placed parts of the motor pathways, notably the internal capsule. The internal capsule is a narrow region of white matter through which the neurons from the motor cortex pass on their way to the brainstem and spinal cord. In this patient the loss of power in the face, upper limb and the lower limb indicate that the lesion was in the internal capsule.

BIBLIOGRAPHY

Axford J, O'Callaghan C. 2004. *Medicine*, 2nd edn. Oxford: Blackwell.

Fitzgerald M J T, Hruener G, Mtui E. 2007. *Clinical Neuroanatomy and Neuroscience*. Philadelphia: Elsevier Saunders.

Kiernan J A. 2005. *Barr's The Human Nervous System: An Anatomical Viewpoint*, 8th edn. Philadelphia: Lippincott Williams and Wilkins.

Kumar P, Clark M. 2005. *Clinical Medicine*, 6th edn. Edinburgh: Elsevier Saunders.

[a]Christian Doppler (1803–1853), Austrian mathematician and physicist, who described the Doppler effect, the apparent change in frequency and wavelength of a wave as perceived by an observer moving relative to the source of the wave.

NEUROLOGY

NEUROLOGY
3. MULTIPLE SCLEROSIS

You are a GP waiting on your final patient on a busy Friday afternoon. You check the computer screen and see that it is a 28-year-old woman, Miss Fraser. You are well acquainted with Miss Fraser as she has been attending your practice frequently over the past few months following a diagnosis of multiple sclerosis.

Multiple sclerosis is a disease characterised by demyelination of the neurons within the central nervous system (CNS).

Q 1. Which cells are responsible for myelin production in the CNS and in the peripheral nervous system (PNS)? *1 mark*

CNS: oligodendrocytes (½ mark).

PNS: Schwann cells (½ mark).

Q 2. Label this diagram of a neuron (Figure 6.6). *3 marks*

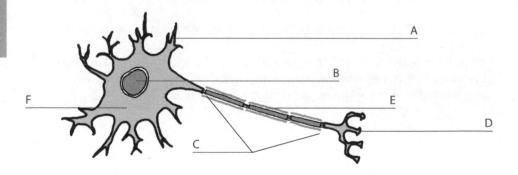

Figure 6.6: A neuron.

A ½ mark for each of the following:

A – Dendrites.

B – Nucleus.

C – Axon.

D – Bouton (foot).

E – Myelin sheath.

F – Soma (body).

Q **3. Give three ways in which a (lower) motor neuron differs from a sensory neuron.** *3 marks*

A 1 mark for any of the following differences:

A Motor neuron:

- all myelinated
- transmission from CNS to muscle fibres
- multipolar
- cell body in anterior grey horn

A Sensory neuron:

- some myelinated
- transmission to CNS from surroundings
- unipolar
- cell body in dorsal root ganglion

When you last saw Miss Fraser she had been complaining of reduced vision and pain in her right eye. During your examination at the time, you noted that her right pupil was constricting further when you shone a light into her left eye than when you shone light into the right eye directly.

Q **4. What is the name of this phenomenon?** *1 mark*

A Relative afferent pupillary defect.

Q **5. Describe the steps of the normal pupillary light reflex when a light is shone into the eye.** *3 marks*

A ½ mark for each point:

- Light shone into the eye activates retinal ganglion cells.

- This triggers an action potential in the optic nerve.

- Impulse synapses at the pretectal nucleus of the midbrain.

- Passes to Edinger–Westphal (parasympathetic) nucleus of CN III.

- Oculomotor parasympathetic nerve fibres synapse in ciliary ganglion.

- Ciliary ganglion neurons innervate constrictor muscle of iris leading to pupillary constriction.

🗁 LEARNING POINT

The autonomic motor nucleus for the constrictor pupillae muscle, and also for the ciliary muscle, is the Edinger–Westphal nucleus. It lies in the midbrain. The direct and consensual light reflexes are both mediated through this nucleus, as is the accommodation reflex which involves the ciliary as well as the constrictor pupillae muscle. The direct light reflex is a reflex pupillary constriction when light is shone into that eye. The consensual light reflex is a pupillary constriction when light is shone into the opposite eye.

This time, Miss Fraser enters the room and sits down. She tells you that her eye pain has now gone.

'I don't understand doctor, I thought multiple sclerosis was a progressive illness, how can my eyes get better?' You explain to Miss Fraser that this is due to the type of MS she has.

NEUROLOGY

Q 6. Explain three of the different forms of multiple sclerosis.   *3 marks*

A ½ mark for any three of the following types and ½ mark for each explanation:

A Relapsing and remitting

- Demyelination occurs in different parts of the CNS at different times with complete or partial resolution within a few weeks

A Primary progressive

- There is a progressive deterioration of function with little or no remission and cumulative disability

A Secondary progressive

- Disease starts with a relapsing and remitting picture but recovery from each successive relapse becomes less and less complete, causing residual disability

A Fulminant

- Occasionally the condition runs a fulminating severe course over several months

---

📁 LEARNING POINT

Symptoms in multiple sclerosis are variable and characteristically evolve over a period of days before resolving either partially or completely within weeks. Symptoms result from axonal demyelination, which leads to slowing or blockade of conduction. The regression of symptoms is attributed to the resolution of inflammatory oedema and to partial remyelination

NEUROLOGY

Unfortunately, Miss Fraser has not been doing so well. She tells you that she has noticed weakness of her legs and feels like she always needs to use the bathroom. She asks you if this could be due to her MS. You explain that MS commonly involves the spinal cord and the symptoms she is describing are indicative of this.

Q 7. What is the name given to spinal cord involvement in multiple sclerosis?   *1 mark*

A Transverse myelitis (1 mark) (inflammation of the spinal cord gets ½ mark).

Q 8. What clinical signs indicate that multiple sclerosis is affecting the spinal cord?   *3 marks*

A Any three of the following (1 mark each):

- Signs of upper motor neuron lesions (see later).

- Sensory disturbance.

- L'Hermitte's sign – electrical 'buzzing' or shock-like sensations in the limbs and body brought on by movement of the neck.

- Incontinence.

📁 LEARNING POINT

Demyelination in multiple sclerosis has a predilection for the optic nerve, brainstem, cerebellum and spinal cord.

Q 9. Label the following features on this diagram (Figure 6.7) of a sagittal section through the brainstem and cerebellum.

3 marks (½ mark for each item)

Cerebral aqueduct

Cerebellar tonsil

Fourth ventricle

Pons

Medulla oblongata

White matter of the cerebellum

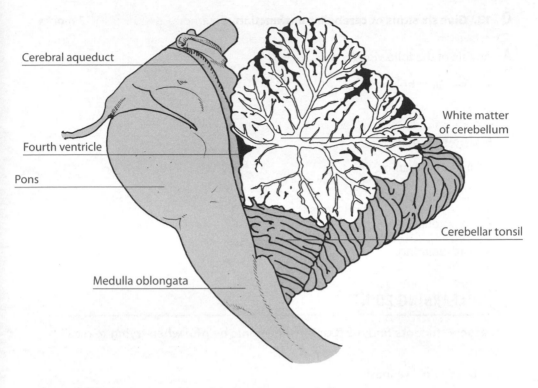

Cerebral aqueduct

White matter
of cerebellum

Fourth ventricle

Pons

Cerebellar tonsil

Medulla oblongata

Figure 6.7: Sagittal section through brainstem and cerebellum.

Q 10. Name the ridges on the surface of the cerebellum. *1 mark*

A Folia.

Q 11. Name the principal nucleus that lies within the cerebellar hemisphere. *1 mark*

A Dentate nucleus.

Q 12. Name the bundles that connect the cerebellum to the midbrain, the pons and the medulla respectively. *1 mark*

A The superior, middle and inferior cerebellar peduncles (1 mark for all 3 in order).

Q 13. **Give six signs of cerebellar dysfunction.**   *3 marks*

A Any six of the following (½ mark for each):

- Dysdiadochokinesis.

- Ataxia.

- Nystagmus.

- Intention tremor.

- Scanning speech.

- Hypotonia.

- Past-pointing.

📁 LEARNING POINT

Glasgow students find the 'Danish' mnemonic helpful when trying to recall these:

D – Dysdiadochokinesis

A – Ataxia

N – Nystagmus (worse looking to the side of the lesion)

I – Intention tremor

S – Scanning speech

H – Hypotonia

It omits the **past-pointing**, however. Better to think of **Danish** Pastry!

Q 14. **What hospital investigation would confirm your suspicions of cerebellar involvement? What would you expect to see?**   *1 mark*

A MRI (½ mark).

A White plaques on cerebellum due to demyelination (½ mark).

📁 LEARNING POINT

An MRI scan is a useful diagnostic and monitoring tool in multiple sclerosis. Demyelination plaques show up white.

Miss Fraser tells you that she has joined a support group for sufferers of MS and that she realises how lucky she is. She tells you that some of the people are wheelchair-bound and unable to move their legs.

You recall that MS affecting the spinal cord can cause an upper motor neuron lesion.

Q 15. **What are the clinical features of an upper motor neuron lesion?** *2 marks*

A Any four of the following (½ mark each):

- Increased muscle tone.
- Spastic paralysis.
- Brisk reflexes.
- Extensor plantar response.
- Clonus.

📖 BIBLIOGRAPHY

Compston A, Confavreux C, Lassmann H, McDonald I R, Miller D H, Noseworthy J, Smith K J, Wekerle H. 2006. *McAlpine's Multiple Sclerosis*, 4th edn. Philadelphia: Churchill Livingstone Elsevier.

Holmes O. 1993. *Human Neurophysiology: A Student Text*, 2nd edn. London: Chapman and Hall Medical.

Kiernan J A. 2005. *Barr's The Human Nervous System: An Anatomical Viewpoint*, 8th edn. Philadelphia: Lippincott Williams and Wilkins.

NEUROLOGY

NEUROLOGY
4. SPINAL CORD COMPRESSION

Miss Hunter is a 38-year-old woman with a known history of breast cancer. She was diagnosed after finding a lump in her right breast 3 years ago. This was identified as a ductal carcinoma-in-situ and was removed with breast conservation, a wide local excision and lymph node dissection. The pathologist reported the cancer as:

- invasive carcinoma, Grade 2, with a maximal diameter of 24 mm
- surgical margins clear of disease
- oestrogen receptor-negative
- metastatic disease in 3 of 16 lymph nodes.

Miss Hunter then underwent radiotherapy and chemotherapy.

Q 1. Mammary glands are specialised accessory glands of the skin. Name four general types of gland associated with the skin. *2 marks*

A ½ mark for each of the following:

- Sudoriferous glands (sweat glands).

- Apocrine glands.

- Sebaceous gland.

- Ceruminous glands (wax-producing glands of the ear).

🗁 LEARNING POINT

Sudoriferous (sweat) glands show merocrine secretion, ie the secretion is released by exocytosis from the apical surface of the cell. Apocrine glands are found in the axilla and perineum and the areola of the breast. They secrete in a similar way to merocrine glands but it is debated whether a small amount of apical cytoplasm is also released. Before the invention of the electron microscope, light microscopy suggested that the apical parts of the cells of apocrine glands separated to form the secretion. Apocrine secretion was believed to occur in the acini of the breast during lactation. If cytoplasm is released with the secretory vacuoles, it is less than initially supposed.

Q **2. Label the following diagram (Figure 6.8) showing the basic structure of the breast.** *3 marks*

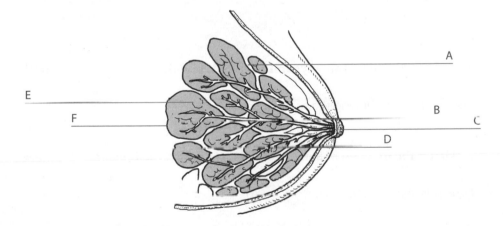

Figure 6.8: Basic anatomy of the breast.

½ mark for each correct label:

A – Suspensory ligament or interlobular connective tissue

B – Lactiferous sinus

C – Nipple

D – Mammary duct

E – Lobule

F – Lobe

After birth, a hormone secreted from the anterior pituitary gland stimulates milk production.

Q **3. What is this hormone called?** *1 mark*

A Prolactin.

Suckling causes the pituitary gland to release oxytocin, which causes the myoepithelial cells to contract.

Q **4. From which part of the pituitary does it come?** *1 mark*

A From posterior pituitary or neurohypophysis.

Q **5. Where is oxytocin produced?** *1 mark*

A Hypothalamus.

Q **6. Where in the breast are myoepithelial cells found?** *1 mark*

A Immediately surrounding the acini.

Q **7. What is the function of a myoepithelial cell within the breast?** *1 mark*

A Contracts to help expel milk.

 LEARNING POINT

Lactation begins after birth when the oestrogen levels fall. This allows prolactin, released from the anterior pituitary, to exert its secretory effect on the mammary glands. Suckling induces the release of oxytocin by the posterior pituitary gland which causes milk ejection.

NEUROLOGY

Miss Hunter has a family history of breast cancer. Her grandmother was diagnosed with breast cancer aged 42. Miss Hunter's mother's elder sister (Miss Hunter's aunt) was diagnosed with breast cancer aged 38. Miss Hunter's elder sister was diagnosed with ovarian cancer last year, aged 42; her younger sister is healthy aged 36. Miss Hunter's mother has not had any cancer and is still healthy aged 66. There is no history of breast or ovarian cancer on Miss Hunter's father's side of the family.

Q **8. Please draw a family tree illustrating Miss Hunter's relevant family history, indicating the age at diagnosis of those individuals affected.** *3 marks*

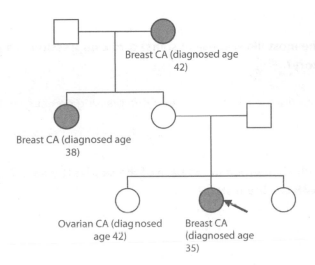

A 1 mark for each of the following:

- Correct family tree structure.

- Correct use of shading to indicate individuals diagnosed with breast cancer.

- Labelling of sister with ovarian cancer (½ mark) but no shading (½ mark).

Q **9. Which two genes are most strongly associated with *both* breast and ovarian cancer?** *1 mark*

A BRCA1 and BRCA2.

LEARNING POINT

Approximately 10% of breast cancer in western countries is thought to have a genetic link.

Three years later, Miss Hunter has now presented to you, her GP, with a 24-hour history of back pain. She has no history of recent injury. She has been feeling lethargic and has lost 3 kg over the last month. You notice as she walks into your surgery that she appears to have an ataxic gait. You are concerned that this could be the start of spinal cord compression and send Jane straight to hospital for urgent assessment.

Q 10. What is the most likely cause of spinal cord compression in a patient with this history? *1 mark*

A Metastatic bone disease (½ mark) in a vertebra pressing on her spinal cord (½ mark).

Q 11. Through which opening in the base of the skull is the spinal cord continuous with the brain stem? *1 mark*

A Foramen magnum.

Q 12. At what vertebral level does the spinal cord end? *1 mark*

A L1–L2 (answers within this range accepted).

Q 13. What is the name of the collection of nerve roots that continue down in the lumbar region of the spinal canal? *1 mark*

A Cauda equina.

NEUROLOGY

Q 14. Below is a diagram (Figure 6.9) of a thoracic vertebra. Identify A–F.

3 marks

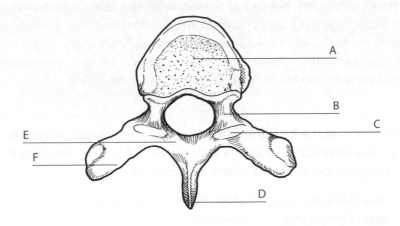

Figure 6.9: The thoracic vertebra.

A ½ mark for each correct label:

A – Vertebral body

B – Pedicle

C – Superior articular process

D – Spinous process

E – Lamina

F – Transverse process

Q 15. At each spinal level, a pair of spinal nerves emerges from the intervertebral foramina. What connects each of these spinal nerves to the spinal cord?

1 mark

A Dorsal root (½ mark) and ventral root (½ mark).

LEARNING POINT

The dorsal (posterior) root carries sensory (afferent) fibres, and the ventral (anterior) root carries motor (efferent) fibres. The dorsal root ganglion is situated on the dorsal root within the intervertebral foramen. This is where the cell bodies of the sensory fibres of the nerve are located. Immediately beyond the ganglion the roots unite to form the spinal nerve.

Jane arrives at the hospital where the receiving doctor agrees a diagnosis of spinal cord compression is possible. He conducts a neurological examination which now shows:

- loss of vibration sense below the level of the umbilicus
- loss of proprioception at the toes
- bilateral lower limb weakness with a 3/5 degree of severity in flexors and extensors of the thighs, legs and feet.

The loss of vibration and proprioception sense might indicate compression of a particular region of the spinal cord.

Q **16. On the diagram below (Figure 6.10), please shade the area of the tracts whose compression is most likely to cause loss of vibration and proprioception.** *1 mark*

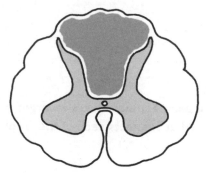

Figure 6.10: Transverse section of spinal cord

NEUROLOGY

Q **17. Loss of vibration sensation below the level of the umbilicus would indicate a spinal cord compression at what spinal level?** *1 mark*

A T10.

Q **18. Please fill in the table below.** *6 marks*

Pathway	Ascending/descending?	What modalities/functions are mediated via the pathway?
Lateral corticospinal tract	Descending (½ mark)	Skilled voluntary movement (½ mark)
Dorsal column/medial lemniscus pathway	Ascending (½ mark)	Fine touch (½ mark), Proprioception (½ mark)
Spinothalamic tract	Ascending (½ mark)	Pain (½ mark), temperature (½ mark), coarse touch (½ mark), pressure (½ mark)
Spinocerebellar tract	Ascending (½ mark)	Muscle and joint receptors (½ mark)

Spinal cord compression is an oncological emergency and a steroid therapy was started and imaging arranged to assess the appropriateness of surgery and radiotherapy in treatment.

NEUROLOGY

📖 BIBLIOGRAPHY

Fitzgerald M J T, Hruener G, Mtui E. 2007. *Clinical Neuroanatomy and Neuroscience*. Philadelphia: Elsevier Saunders.

Kiernan J A. 2005. *Barr's The Human Nervous System: An Anatomical Viewpoint*, 8th edn. Philadelphia: Lippincott Williams and Wilkins.

Nussbaum R L, McInnes R R, Willard H F. 2007. *Genetics in Medicine*, 7th edn. Philadelphia: Saunders.

NEUROLOGY
5. STROKE

Mr McKay is a 68-year-old man who is attending a routine check up at his local GP practice. He has no symptoms and urine dipstick test is negative. His blood pressure is 155/98 mmHg and he has a body mass index (BMI) of 30 kg/m^2.

Q 1. How do you routinely measure systolic and diastolic blood pressure using a stethoscope?   *2 marks*

A Take measurements using a sphygmomanometer. Place the inflatable cuff round the arm. Inflate the cuff until pressure is greater than that expected. Slowly deflate the cuff with stethoscope over the brachial artery. Systolic pressure is when Korotkoff's[a] sounds are first heard (1 mark). Diastolic pressure is when the Korotkoff's sounds become muffled (1 mark).

Q 2. Prior to treatment, what would you do next with regard to this blood pressure result?   *1 mark*

A Record the reading in the notes and arrange for two repeat measurements at separate times (½ mark) and give lifestyle advice (½ mark).

Q 3. What is the equation for calculating mean arterial pressure from the measured pressures?   *1 mark*

A MAP= DP + (PP/3), where MAP is mean arterial pressure, DP is diastolic pressure and PP is pulse pressure.

A NB. Pulse pressure = systolic blood pressure – diastolic blood pressure.

📁 LEARNING POINT

The MAP is a time-weighted average of the arterial pressure over the whole of the cardiac cycle. It is not a simple average of the diastolic and systolic pressures. This is because the arterial blood spends much longer near the diastolic pressure level than near the systolic. The MAP also has a relationship with cardiac output (CO) and the total peripheral resistance (TPR), MAP = CO×TPR, but this is not what this question was looking for.

Q 4. How is body mass index calculated? *1 mark*

A BMI = mass (kg)/[height (m)]^2.

Q 5. Into what body mass index category would the following patients fall? *1 mark*

Q 5(a). A man with BMI index = 15.0 kg/m^2.

Q 5(b). A woman with BMI = 35.0 kg/m^2.

A (a) Underweight (½ mark).

A (b) Obese (½ mark).

📁 LEARNING POINT

The boundaries for the categories vary somewhat between centres. The following are commonly used:

<18.5 kg/m^2	= underweight
18.5–24.9 kg/m^2	= normal weight
25–29.9 kg/m^2	= overweight
≥30 kg/m^2	= obese

NEUROLOGY

The GP later decides to treat Mr McKay's raised blood pressure. Mr McKay is unhappy, however, as he feels fit and healthy and asks why he is being put on medication when he feels well.

Q 6. Suggest three advantages/reasons for Mr McKay being put on medication to control his hypertension.   *2 marks*

A Decreases risk of/or prevents stroke (½ mark), ischaemic heart disease (½ mark), renal failure (1 mark).

Q 7. Give three classes of drug commonly used in the treatment of hypertension. For each class, briefly describe their mechanism of action.   *6 marks*

A 1 mark for each class of drug and for its mechanism:

Type of drug	Mechanism of action
Diuretics	Reduces blood volume by inhibiting electrolyte transport in the renal tubules
ACE inhibitors	Inhibition of angiotensin converting enzyme (ACE), which reduces angiotensin II and aldosterone levels. This causes vasodilatation with reduction in peripheral resistance
Calcium-channel blockers	Relaxes vascular smooth muscle decreasing peripheral vascular resistance

Mr McKay is concerned about the side-effects. He describes having a friend who is on treatment for hypertension and suffers from dizzy spells when standing up. This is postural hypotension.

Q 8. When a healthy person stands up what physiological mechanism maintains/restores blood pressure?   *2 marks*

A When the blood pressure falls the rate of discharge of the baroreceptors (½ mark) in the aortic arch (½ mark) and in the carotid sinus (½ mark) decreases and gives rise to an increase (½ mark) in sympathetic (½ mark) discharge to the heart and vasculature. Cardiac output is increased and there is a rise in total peripheral resistance. These both maintain/restore normal blood pressure.

Q **9. Explain the physiological mechanism by which postural hypotension occurs.** *1½ marks*

A When a person stands up quickly, there is a sudden fall in venous return to the heart from the veins of the lower limbs (½ mark). This leads to a fall in stroke volume (by Starling's law) (½ mark), cardiac output (½ mark) and therefore blood pressure.

Q **10. In a healthy young adult, which is more noticeable on moving from a lying to a standing position – a fall in blood pressure or a rise in heart rate?** *½ mark*

A In a healthy young adult the physiological mechanism that maintains blood pressure is so efficient that there is minimal fall in blood pressure but a rise in heart rate.

📁 **LEARNING POINT**

The increase in heart rate on standing is largely due to a reduction in vagal tone.

Several weeks later you are called by Mr McKay's wife who came home and found him collapsed on the floor. He is very confused and his speech sounds abnormal. He also has an obvious weakness on the right side of his body. You suspect he has had a stroke.

You note that Mr McKay has an irregular pulse. Upon further examination you find he has trouble comprehending spoken and written language, producing coherent speech, and has paralysis on the right side in his upper limb and face but not in his lower limb.

NEUROLOGY

Q 11. What are the two specific areas in the brain concerned with speech and what language problems can result from damage to these areas? *2 marks*

A Broca's[b] area – coordinates speech production (½ mark). Damage gives expressive aphasia (½ mark).

A Wernicke's[c] area – centre for comprehension of speech (½ mark). Damage gives receptive aphasia (½ mark).

Q 12. Identify A–H on the diagram (Figure 6.11) of the circle of Willis[d] and the major arteries supplying the brain. *4 marks*

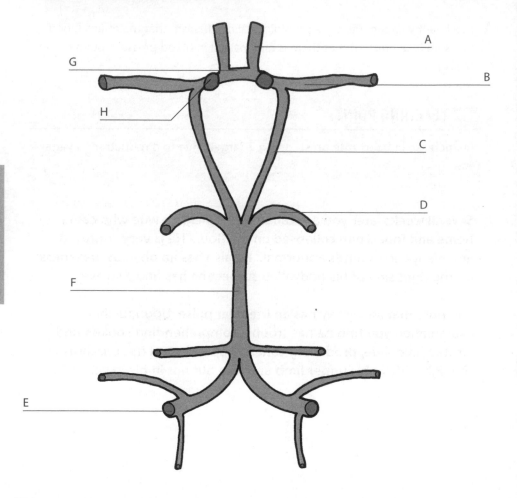

Figure 6.11: Circle of Willis.

A ½ mark for each artery:

A – Anterior cerebral artery

B – Middle cerebral artery

C – Posterior communicating artery

D – Posterior cerebral artery

E – Vertebral artery

F – Basilar artery

G – Anterior communicating artery

H – Internal carotid artery

Q **13. Blockage of which artery is most likely to explain this man's symptoms?**   *1 mark*

A Left middle cerebral artery.

📁 **LEARNING POINT**

Broca's and Wernicke's areas for speech and language are normally situated on the side of the brain that controls the dominant upper limb and are both supplied by the middle cerebral artery. Most people are right-handed so the dominant side of the brain is the left, the motor pathways being crossed. Thus, since Mr McKay has paralysis of his right upper limb and speech deficits, it is reasonable to assume his stroke has occurred in the left side of his brain and that he is right-handed. The right lower limb is unaffected. The region of the motor cortex that controls the lower limb is more superiorly placed and receives its blood from the anterior cerebral artery.

Mr McKay arrives in hospital. A CT scan of his brain shows an area of ischaemia in the regions of the left hemisphere adjacent to the lateral fissure, and an ECG shows atrial fibrillation (AF).

Q 14. On the following diagram (Figure 6.12) indicate the territories of the cerebral arteries.   *3 marks*

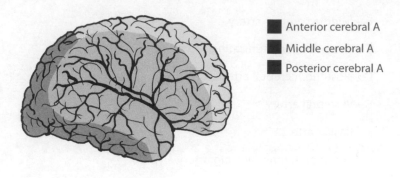

■ Anterior cerebral A

■ Middle cerebral A

■ Posterior cerebral A

Figure 6.12: Territories of the cerebral arteries.

A (1 mark for accurate representation of the territory supplied by each cerebral artery)

Q 15. Of the clinical information gathered on the patient to date, what is the most likely explanation of why he has had a stroke?   *2 marks*

A Atrial fibrillation is a well-recognised complication of hypertension (1 mark) resulting from its deleterious effect on the heart. The disordered functioning of the atria means that blood is not pumped effectively through the atria and can consequently clot (1 mark) and lead to embolism. An embolus has lodged in the left middle cerebral artery.

🗁 LEARNING POINT

Students may wonder whether the high blood pressure has ruptured an artery in the brain and/or caused an internal capsule lesion. Haemorrhage from an artery would probably have been seen on the scan. A lesion of the internal capsule would probably have caused paralysis of the lower limb on the same side as the paralysis of the upper limb and face.

📖 BIBLIOGRAPHY

Axford J, O'Callaghan C. 2004. *Medicine*, 2nd edn. Oxford: Blackwell.

Fitzgerald M J T, Hruener G, Mtui E. 2007. *Clinical Neuroanatomy and Neuroscience*. Philadelphia: Elsevier Saunders.

Kiernan J A. 2005. *Barr's The Human Nervous System: An Anatomical Viewpoint*, 8th edn. Philadelphia: Lippincott Williams and Wilkins.

Widmaier E P, Roff H, Strang K T. 2006. *Vander's Human Physiology. The Mechanism of Body Function*, 10th edn. Boston: McGraw Hill.

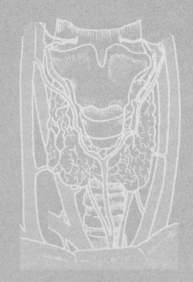

ENDOCRINOLOGY CASES:
ANSWERS

ENDOCRINOLOGY
1. ADDISON'S DISEASE

You are a junior doctor in Accident and Emergency when one Saturday morning 58-year-old Mr Gordon is rushed in. He was found by his wife, who has followed the ambulance to the hospital. She is very anxious and struggles to give a clear history. Mr Gordon has reduced consciousness and appears to be seriously unwell.

You begin an initial assessment and discover that Mr Gordon is cold and clammy with a blood pressure of 90/60 mmHg and a heart rate of 140 beats per minute, leading you to consider that he might be in shock.

As you begin a more thorough examination, you discover a silver bracelet (Figure 7.1) around his wrist with the following symbol.

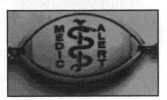

On noticing this you question Mrs Gordon about her husband's medical history and medication, and discover that he was diagnosed with Addison's disease[a] 5 months ago and started on daily corticosteroid replacement therapy.

Figure 7.1

Q 1. What is Addison's disease? *1 mark*

A Addison's disease is chronic adrenal insufficiency (1 mark) due to destruction of the adrenal cortex.

Addison's disease is relatively rare: with a prevalence of about 4 per 100 000 people in the UK.

Q **2. What is the main aetiology in affluent countries?** *1 mark*

A Autoimmune adrenalitis.

 LEARNING POINT

In developing countries tuberculosis is the commonest cause

Mrs Gordon also tells you that a fortnight ago her husband was an in-patient and was diagnosed with severe community-acquired pneumonia, and treated with amoxicillin.

His respiratory symptoms have now subsided, but over the last few days he has been vomiting and has been 'off his food'. His temperature has been around 38°C, and he has been complaining of generalised abdominal pain, weakness and dizziness, especially when he tries to stand. Mrs Gordon has also noticed a change in mood, her husband having become somewhat apathetic. More worryingly, he has become acutely confused within the last 24 hours.

Q **3. What drug would you administer now and how?** *2 marks*

A Give an intravenous (1 mark) bolus of hydrocortisone (1 mark).

The next morning a short synacthen test was performed:

Mr Gordon's results:

Time (min)	Cortisol level in Mr Gordon's serum (nmol/l)	Normal serum levels throughout test (nmol/l)
0	90	> 170
30	90	> 580

Q **4. Explain Mr Gordon's low baseline serum cortisol level (time 0) and why his body does not respond to the synacthen test (+ 30 min).** *2 marks*

A Mr Gordon has a low basal cortisol level as his body is using it at a greater rate than normal (due to infection) but he has not increased his dosage to account for this. His basal level has thus fallen (1 mark).

A His 30-min cortisol level does not rise as there is significant adrenal atrophy due to his Addison's disease (1 mark).

🗁 LEARNING POINT

The short synacthen test is performed to test the adrenal reserve:
- Take a basal serum level of cortisol
- Give 250 µg of synacthen (synthetic ACTH) intravenously at time 0
- Measure blood cortisol levels at time +30, +60 min

In healthy individuals, the basal plasma cortisol should exceed 170 nmol/l and rise to at least 580 nmol/l. The hypoadrenal patient is unable to raise their serum cortisol in response to synacthen.

The adrenals (suprarenals) are endocrine glands located at the superior poles of the kidneys. The left is crescentic and the right tetrahedral in shape.

Q **5. Identify A–C in the diagram below (Figure 7.2).** *1 mark*

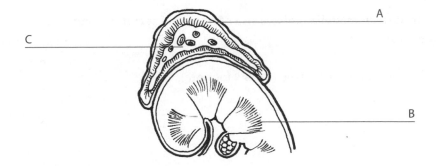

Figure 7.2: Adrenal gland.

A – Adrenal cortex (½ mark).

B – Kidney.

C – Adrenal medulla (½ mark).

🗁 LEARNING POINT

The adrenal and kidney are often separated by a layer of adipose tissue. On magnetic resonance imaging the fat is seen as a light gap between the two organs.

Q 6. Name the three zones of the adrenal cortex and the hormone produced from each of these areas.   *3 marks*

Zone of adrenal cortex	Hormone
Zone glomerulosa (½ mark)	Aldosterone/mineralocorticoid (½ mark)
Zona fasciculata (½ mark) and zona reticularis (½ mark)	Cortisol/glucocorticoid (½ mark) and adrenal androgen (½ mark)

🗁 LEARNING POINT

Cortisol and adrenal androgen are thought to be produced by both the zona fasciculata and the zona reticularis.

Q 7. The adrenal medulla is also a site of hormone secretion: name its products.   *1 mark*

A Adrenaline and noradrenaline (1 mark for both).

Q **8. Complete the diagram (Figure 7.3) below illustrating the homeostatic control of cortisol release.**   *3 marks*

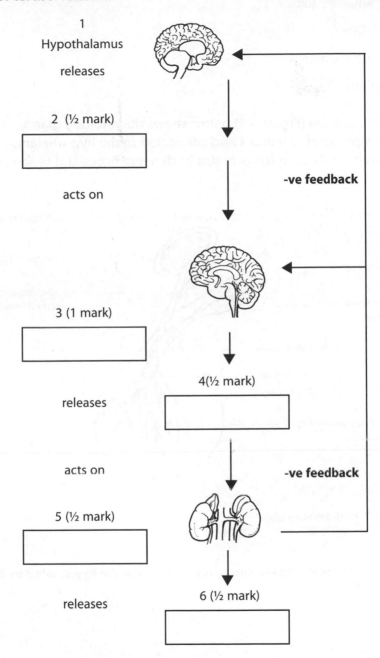

Figure 7.3: Homeostatic control of cortisol release.

A 2. CRH (corticotrophin releasing hormone)

   3. Anterior pituitary

   4. ACTH

   5. Adrenal glands

   6. Cortisol

The diagram (Figure 7.4) below shows the pituitary gland, composed of two lobes and connected to the hypothalamus by the pituitary stalk, which contains both nerve fibres and blood vessels.

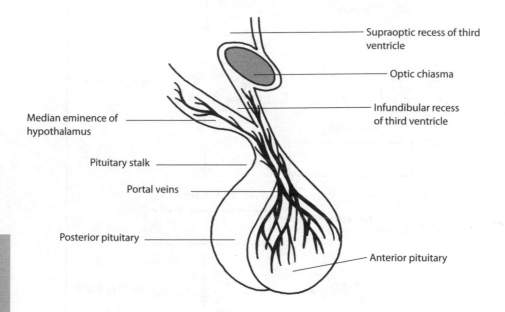

Figure 7.4: The pituitary gland.

Q 9. **Which lobe of the pituitary is connected to the hypothalamus by blood vessels?**   *1 mark*

A Anterior lobe.

Q 10. Name these vessels. *1 mark*

A Hypophysial portal veins.

Q 11. Which hormones travel to the pituitary gland via nerve fibres? *1 mark*

A Oxytocin (½ mark) and antidiuretic hormone (½ mark).

Q 12. Which hormones are produced by the anterior pituitary? *3 marks*

A ½ mark for each of the following:

- Adrenocorticotrophic hormone (ACTH)
- Follicle-stimulating hormone
- Growth hormone
- Luteinising hormone
- Prolactin
- Thyroid-stimulating hormone

📁 LEARNING POINT

Melanocyte-stimulating hormone is produced by the intermediate lobe, in humans a thin layer of cells between the anterior and posterior lobes. To avoid this being a problem, it is probably better to refer to the adenohypophysis (anterior and intermediate lobes) and the neurohypophysis (posterior lobe).

ENDOCRINOLOGY

Q **13. What are the main effects of cortisol in the body?**   *3 marks*

A Metabolic (½ mark each for any two of the following):

- Stimulates gluconeogenesis

- Glycogenesis

- Lipolysis

- Opposes insulin (raises blood glucose level)

A Immunosuppression (½ mark each for any two of the following):

- Decreases lymphoid tissue (volume and activity): ↓antibodies, ↓ lymphocytes

- Anti-inflammatory (blocks recruitment of eosinophils, interleukins-1, -2 and -6 plus tumour necrosis factor)

A Systemic (½ mark each for any two of the following):

- Increased appetite

- ↓ Vitamin D3 and therefore calcium absorption

- ↑ Bone resorption

- Promotes the effects of adrenaline therefore increased vascular tone/blood pressure

🗁 LEARNING POINT

Steroid hormones, such as cortisol, oestradiol and testosterone are hydrophobic signal molecules that pass through the plasma membrane of their target cells. Thyroxine is chemically an amine but it acts like a steroid. Once inside the cell these hormones bind to receptor proteins located in either the cytosol or the nucleus. When a hormone binds, the receptor protein undergoes a large conformational change that activates the protein, allowing it to promote or inhibit the transcription of a selected set of genes and therefore stimulate the desired response from the cell.

ENDOCRINOLOGY

Q 14. Using the diagram from Question 8 explain how taking daily oral corticosteroids affects the normal production of hormones from all layers in the adrenal glands. *2 marks*

A Corticosteroid use increases the concentration of cortisol in the body. This increases the negative feedback (½ mark) on the hypothalamus and the anterior pituitary and thus in turn decreases the production of CRH (corticotrophin releasing hormone) (½ mark) and ACTH (½ mark). Due to the decreasing levels of ACTH, there is under-stimulation of the adrenal glands and they atrophy (½ mark).

📁 LEARNING POINT

This atrophy means that the glands no longer produce such high levels of (or, if atrophy is extensive, any) hormones and, therefore, supplementation of both glucocorticoids (cortisol) and mineralocorticoids (aldosterone) is a necessity. If steroid treatment is to be stopped, it must always be done slowly and carefully.

Mr Gordon's hospital case notes have now arrived. Prior to his initial diagnosis of Addison's disease, he had experienced loss of appetite, nausea, occasional vomiting and weight loss. He felt weak and somewhat depressed and complained of being suddenly dizzy on standing up. Moreover he had noticed patches of dull/grey discoloration appearing mainly on areas exposed to both light and pressure: his elbows, knuckles, palmar creases, and also on a recent scar on his left knee

Q 15. Explain the cause of these pigmentation patches. *1 mark*

A In primary hypoadrenalism there is increased ACTH secretion (½ mark) from the anterior pituitary to try to stimulate more cortisol production. However, ACTH contains a sequence similar to melanocyte-stimulating hormone (½ mark), which causes pigmentation of the skin and buccal surfaces when ACTH levels are very high.

Q **16. In which layer of the skin are the melanocytes found?** *1 mark*

A Basal layer of the epidermis (stratum basale) (1 mark) and underlying dermis.

The next day the results of Mr Gordon's blood tests taken on admission become available.

	Mr Gordon's serum levels	**Normal range**
Na⁺	80 mmol/l	135–145 mmol/l
K⁺	6.7 mmol/l	3.5–5.0 mmol/l
Blood glucose (fasting)	2.5 mmol/l	3.5–5.5 mmol/l
Urea	18.0 mmol/l	2.5–6.7 mmol/l
Creatinine	178 µmol/l	70–150 µmol/l

Q **17. Explain these biochemical abnormalities.** *2 marks*

- *Hyponatraemia* – mineralocorticoid deficiency (↓ aldosterone), therefore sodium depletion (plus reduced extracellular fluid and hypotension) (½ mark)

- *Hyperkalaemia* – reduced renal K^+ excretion (as aldosterone normally increases K^+ excretion alongside Na^+ reabsorption) (½ mark)

- *Hypoglycaemia* – from reduced glycogen stores (cortisol normally ↑ gluconeogenesis and glycogenesis) (½ mark)

- ↑ *Urea:creatinine ratio* – signs of dehydration (½ mark)

Mr Gordon is also taking 75 µg fludrocortisone twice daily.

Q **18. What is this drug and why is it important in the treatment of Addison's disease?** *1 mark*

A A mineralocorticoid replacement (½ mark).

A It is necessary to replace the normal mineralocorticoid that is suppressed in Addison's disease (½ mark).

After 48 h Mr Gordon has been stabilised and is moved to the medical ward for monitoring until he is fit to go home.

On discharge you warn Mr and Mrs Gordon again about the seriousness of this situation, and how lucky he has been on this occasion. Careful attention must be given to avoid a similar episode happening again and he must always remember to wear his 'Medic Alert' bracelet.

📖 BIBLIOGRAPHY

Besser G M, Thorner M O. 2002. *Comprehensive Clinical Endocrinology*, 3rd edn. London: Mosby.

Greenspan F S, Stewler G J. 1997. *Basic and Clinical Endocrinology*, 5th edn. London: Prentice Hall.

[a]Thomas Addison (1793–1860). An Edinburgh graduate (1815), Addison became a physician and lecturer in Materia Medica at Guy's Hospital, London, where he was a skilful diagnostician. He committed suicide at the age of 67, having been forced to retire because of melancholia.

ENDOCRINOLOGY
2. DIABETES MELLITUS

You are the receiving physician in the Accident and Emergency Department. Miss Winters is a 23-year-old engineering student who presents drowsy and confused. Her sister has brought her in and tells you that Miss Winters has been an insulin-dependent diabetic since childhood. For the past 2 days Miss Winters has had 'food poisoning'. Miss Winters's heart rate is 116 beats per minute and her blood pressure is 95/60 mmHg. There is reduced skin turgor and her tongue is dry.

Q 1. Which cells secrete insulin and to which group of cells in the pancreas do they belong? *1 mark*

A Beta/β cells (½ mark) of the pancreatic islets (½ mark) (of Langerhans[a]).

🗁 LEARNING POINT

The endocrine cells of the pancreas are arranged into groups known as pancreatic islets. They are scattered throughout the pancreas but are more numerous in the body and tail. Alpha/α cells secrete glucagon, beta/β cells secrete insulin, delta/δ cells secrete somatostatin (growth hormone inhibiting hormone) and PP/F cells secrete pancreatic polypeptide.

Q 2. Precisely how do the cells that secrete insulin react to increasing concentrations of circulating glucose? *3 marks*

A Glucose enters β cells via GLUT-2 receptors (½ mark).

A It is metabolised and ATP is produced (½ mark).

A This inhibits ATP-sensitive K⁺ channels, preventing K⁺ efflux (½ mark).

A This causes depolarisation of the cell (½ mark) and Ca^{2+} influx is increased (½ mark). Increasing Ca^{2+} causes insulin to be secreted (½ mark).

Q 3. What is the general structure of the human insulin molecule in the bloodstream? *1 mark*

A Insulin consists of two polypeptide chains linked by disulphide bonds.

Q 4. What protein, secreted with insulin, can be used as a marker for insulin production? *1 mark*

A C-peptide.

 LEARNING POINT

Insulin is synthesised as one long polypeptide chain. The cleaving of C-peptide from the chain produces the two-subunit structure.

Q 5. Describe the transduction of the insulin signal in the effector cell. *4 marks*

A Any four of the following:

- Insulin receptor has alpha and beta subunits (1 mark).
- Binding of insulin to the receptor causes autophosphorylation of the beta unit (1 mark).
- Autophosphorylation causes tyrosine kinase activation (1 mark).
- Enzyme cascades are activated (1 mark) including phosphoinositide-3-kinase (1 mark).
- GLUT-4 receptors are translocated to the cell membrane (1 mark).
- Glucose enters the cell via the GLUT-4 receptor (1 mark).

ENDOCRINOLOGY

📁 LEARNING POINT

Glucose enters the glycolysis pathway when it enters the cell. The first stage in this pathway is the formation of glucose-6 phosphate. This reaction is controlled by the hexokinase enzyme. Most hexokinases have very high affinities for glucose relative to the level in the blood. They are half-saturated at concentrations of less than 0.1 mmol/l and the normal blood glucose concentration is 4–5 mmol/l. These hexokinases are also product inhibited.

Hepatocytes contain a hexokinase isoenzyme known as glucokinase which has a much lower affinity for glucose and does not become saturated. It is product-inhibited at concentrations outside the normal physiological range and so produces much more glucose-6 phosphate than the other hexokinases. The large amount of glucose-6 phosphate produced is used to form glycogen, the glucose storage molecule.

By producing glucose-6-phosphate, the glucose cannot leave the cell and a concentration gradient for glucose entry into the cell is maintained.

Q **6. Is Miss Winters likely to be a type I or type II diabetic?** *1 mark*

A Type I.

Q **7. Which form of diabetes is usually an HLA-associated autoimmune disease?** *1 mark*

A Type I.

Q **8. What would be an appropriate adjustment to an insulin regime during a period of intercurrent illness and why?** *1 mark*

A Increase the insulin (½ mark). Illness causes an increase in cortisol which counters the action of insulin (½ mark).

Miss Winters is still drowsy and taking deep sighing breaths despite oxygen. A finger-prick sample of blood shows that her glucose level is 25 mmol/l and her urine is positive for ketones and glucose.

Q **9. What is the name given to the hyperventilation that Miss Winters is demonstrating?** *1 mark*

A Kussmaul[b] breathing.

Q **10. Which three ketones are produced during diabetic ketoacidosis?** *1 mark*

A Acetoacetate, β-hydroxybutyrate and acetone.

Q **11. Explain how insulin deficiency results in ketone production.** *3 marks*

A Any six of the following:

- Deficiency of insulin causes excessive lipolysis (½ mark).
- Fatty acids are broken down to acetyl CoA (½ mark).
- Normally acetyl CoA enters the Kreb's[c]/citric acid cycle (½ mark).
- Excess acetyl CoA is converted to acetoacetyl CoA (½ mark).
- Acetoacetyl CoA is metabolised by the liver (½ mark) producing acetoacetate (½ mark) and β-hydroxybutyrate (½ mark).
- Production of ketones exceeds their metabolism (½ mark).

You take an arterial blood gas sample. The results are:

Parameter	Miss Winters' value	Normal range
pH	7.05	7.35–7.45
[H+] (nmol/l)	90	35–45
[HCO$_3^-$] (mmol/l)	8.0	20
pCO_2 (kPa)	2.0	4.7–6

Q **12. What type of acid–base abnormality is shown?** *1 mark*

A Metabolic (½ mark) acidosis (½ mark).

Q **13. Explain how the low $p CO_2$ has occurred.** *2 marks*

A Rise in plasma $[H^+]$ stimulates respiration (1 mark).

A Increased respiration causes decreased levels of CO_2 in blood (1 mark).

A venous blood sample sent for urea and electrolyte analysis gives the following results:

Parameter	Miss Winters' value (mmol/l)	Normal range (mmol/l)
Na	138	135–146
K	5.2	3.5–5.0
Cl	99	98–106
HCO_3	5.4	22–30
Urea	11.2	2.5–6.7
Creatinine	125	89–118

Q **14. What evidence is there that the patient is dehydrated?** *2 marks*

A Any four of the following:

- Dry tongue (½ mark).

- Reduced skin turgor (½ mark).

- Low blood pressure (½ mark).

- Elevated urea (½ mark) with less change in creatinine (½ mark).

📁 LEARNING POINT

Be careful in using a dry tongue to assess dehydration. The patient may simply have been breathing through the mouth!

Q 15. Calculate the anion gap in this patient. *1 mark*

A Anion gap $=([Na^+]+[K^+])-([Cl^-]+[HCO_3^-])$

$=(138+5)-(99+5)=39$ mmol/l.

Q 16. This anion gap is high. What is the normal gap? *1 mark*

A The anion gap is usually <18 mmol/l.

Q 17. Why has this large anion gap resulted in this patient? *1 mark*

A The high anion gap in diabetic ketoacidosis results from accumulation of organic acids.

📂 **LEARNING POINT**

The anion gap provides a means of ascertaining whether the acidosis is due to retention of HCl or another acid. It is based on the principle that the sum of positive and negative charges in the plasma is equal.

If the anion gap is normal, this suggests that HCl is being retained or $NaHCO_3$ is being lost. Under these conditions, plasma bicarbonate decreases but is replaced by chloride to maintain electroneutrality.

If the anion gap is high there are unmeasured anions present in large quantities. This may be a normal acid, eg lactate, which is not normally measured or some other acid such as acetoacetic acid.

Whilst you are waiting for Miss Winters's blood results to return, you start treatment.

Q 18. Which aspect of Miss Winters's condition will you manage first and how? *2 marks*

A Dehydration (1 mark) by giving intravenous saline (½ mark) as quickly as possible (½ mark).

Miss Winters's sister asks why their grandmother, who was only diagnosed with diabetes last year, never has the same problem with her illness that Miss Winters does.

Q 19. What endocrine emergency can occur in type II diabetics? *1 mark*

A Hyperosmolar (½ mark) non-ketotic (½ mark) coma or HONK (½ mark).

Q 20. This condition requires anticoagulation in addition to management of the metabolic emergency. Which drug is used in this purpose? *1 mark*

A Heparin.

 LEARNING POINT

Diabetic ketoacidosis is an emergency that occurs only in type I diabetics. Both ketosis and acidosis need to be present for the diagnosis to be made. The life-threatening nature of diabetic ketoacidosis is due to the dehydration, not the hyperglycaemia, so correcting dehydration is more important. The insulin given depends on the local protocols and sliding scales.

Hyperglycaemic hyperosmolar non-ketotic states (HONK) occur only in type II diabetics. This tends to be a more insidious presentation with marked dehydration and hyperglycaemia. There is no switch to ketone metabolism and therefore there is no acidosis. The hyperosmolar state increases the risk of thrombosis, so anticoagulation must be started.

BIBLIOGRAPHY

Kumar P, Clark M. 2000. *Acute Clinical Medicine*. Sutton, Surrey: Reed Healthcare Publishing.

Kumar P, Clark M. 2005. *Clinical Medicine,* 6th edn. Edinburgh: Elsevier Saunders.

McHardy K C, Godden D J, Nathwani D, Needham G, Duguid K P. 1994. *Illustrated Cases in Acute Clinical Medicine*. Edinburgh: Churchill Livingstone.

Sawyer N, Gabriel R, Gabriel C M. 1989. *300 Medical Data Interpretation Questions for MRCP*, 3rd edn. London: Butterworths.

[a]Paul Langerhans (1847–1888), German pathologist and biologist. He described the pancreatic islets in 1869. He also discovered the Langerhans cells of the epidermis, a form of dendritic cell. Langerhans died of tuberculosis and renal disease in Madeira and was buried in the British Cemetery.

[b]Adolf Kussmaul (1822–1902), German physician. A very precise observer of his patients, who made many classic descriptions, including the pattern of breathing in diabetic ketoacidosis and the effect of obstructive chest disease on the jugular venous pulse.

[c]Hans Adolf Krebs (1900–1981), German and later British clinician and biochemist. He identified the urea cycle in 1932. In 1933, Krebs went to Cambridge where, in 1937, he documented the citric acid cycle for which he was awarded a Nobel Prize in 1953.

ENDOCRINOLOGY

ENDOCRINOLOGY
3. THYROID DISEASE

You are a GP at the University Health Centre. Miss Taylor, a 19-year-old student, comes to see you complaining of having 'a lot of nervous energy'. In the past four months, she has been sweating excessively and has lost 5 kg despite having an increased appetite. She has also been having difficulty concentrating on her studies and is finding the lecture theatres too warm. You notice Miss Taylor has exophthalmos, the upper edge of both corneas being invisible. She also has a tremor and her pulse is 102 beats per minute at rest.

You suspect that Miss Taylor has hyperthyroidism.

Q **1. What is the normal relationship of the upper lid to the cornea?** *1 mark*

A Normally the upper lid crosses the cornea so that the uppermost part of the iris is obscured.

Q **2. Name the thyroid hormones and indicate which is more potent.** *3 marks*

T_3 – tri-iodothyronine (1 mark).

T_4 – thyroxine/tetra-iodothyronine (1 mark).

T_3 is more potent (1 mark).

🗀 LEARNING POINT

T_3 is several times more potent than T_4, but T_4 is secreted in greater amounts. As T_4 circulates through peripheral tissues it is de-iodinated and converted into T_3.

Q **3. One of the main actions of thyroid hormones is to regulate the basal metabolic rate (BMR). Define BMR.** *2 marks*

A The calculated equivalent oxygen consumption (½ mark) or heat production (½ mark) by the body, in a fasting subject (½ mark) at complete rest (½ mark).

Q **4. The diagram (Figure 7.5) below shows a thyroid follicle. Label the parts indicated.** *2 marks*

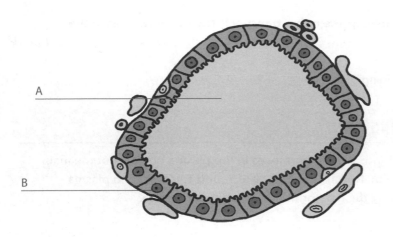

Figure 7.5: A thyroid follicle.

A 1 mark for each of the following:

A – thyroglobulin (or colloid)

B – follicular cells

Q 5. Outline two functions of thyroid follicular cells. *2 marks*

A Any two of the following:

- Transport of iodide from the blood and the trapping of it in the cytosol (iodide trapping) (1 mark).

- Synthesis of thyroglobulin (TGB) (1 mark).

- Resorption of thyroglobulin (1 mark).

- Release of thyroxine from the follicles (1 mark).

Q 6. Name the main protein that transports thyroid hormones in the plasma. *1 mark*

A Thyroxine-binding globulin.

🗁 LEARNING POINT

Albumin also binds thyroid hormones in the plasma but it is not the main transport protein. Normally over 99% of T_3 and T_4 is bound to plasma proteins but only the free forms are metabolically active.

You palpate Miss Taylor's neck and discover that her thyroid gland is enlarged. It is smooth, non-tender and moves upwards with swallowing.

Q **7. Label the diagram below (Figure 7.6).**   *8 marks*

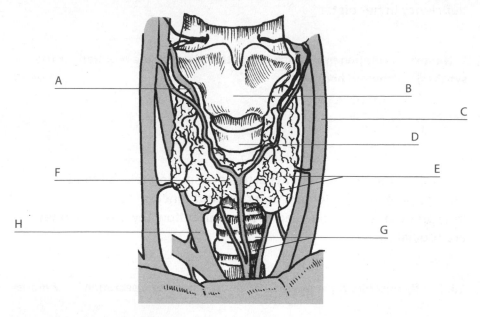

Figure 7.6: Thyroid anatomy.

A 1 mark for each of the following:

A = Superior thyroid artery

B = Thyroid cartilage

C = Internal jugular vein

D = Cricoid cartilage

E = Lobe of thyroid gland

F = Isthmus of the thyroid gland

G = Trachea

H = Common carotid artery

Q **8. Why does the thyroid gland move upwards on swallowing?**   *1 mark*

A The larynx rises on swallowing as the thyroid gland is tethered to it by the pretracheal fascia.

Miss Taylor asks you whether the thyroid enlargement is due to a deficiency in her diet.

Q **9. Name two components derived from the diet that are required for the synthesis of thyroid hormones.** *1 mark*

A Iodine/iodide (½ mark).

Tyrosine (½ mark).

To confirm the diagnosis of hyperthyroidism, you take a blood sample from Miss Taylor and order thyroid function tests. To interpret the results you need to remember how thyroid hormones are regulated.

Q **10. Briefly describe the regulation of thyroid hormone secretion.** *2 marks*

A Thyrotrophin-releasing hormone (TRH) is released from the hypothalamus in response to low T_3 and T_4 levels or low metabolic rate (½ mark).

TRH stimulates the anterior pituitary to release thyroid-stimulating hormone (TSH) (½ mark).

TSH is released into the bloodstream and stimulates thyroid follicular cells to secrete T_3 and T_4 into the bloodstream (½ mark).

Blood levels of T_3 and T_4 reach normal levels and inhibit the release of TRH and TSH (½ mark).

Q **11. What results would you expect from the thyroid function tests to confirm a diagnosis of primary hyperthyroidism?** *1 mark*

A TSH is undetectable (½ mark).

Free T_3 and T_4 are elevated (½ mark).

The tests confirm primary hyperthyroidism and Miss Taylor is prescribed carbimazole. She takes the drug for 24 months but unfortunately experiences recurrent disease one year after stopping

ENDOCRINOLOGY

treatment. She does not want to take radio-iodine treatment and is referred for a surgical opinion. The surgeon recommends a subtotal thyroidectomy (ie partial removal of the thyroid gland) and explains the procedure and some of the complications that sometimes arise.

Q 12. Name the nerves that must be spared during neck surgery to ensure that no voice hoarseness occurs post-operatively. *2 marks*

A Recurrent laryngeal nerve (1 mark) and the external (1 mark) branch of the superior laryngeal nerve.

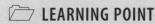

LEARNING POINT

The recurrent laryngeal nerve lies in the groove between the oesophagus and trachea and is closely associated with the inferior thyroid artery. Here it is easily damaged by division, stretching or compression. Damage to one side of the nerve results in hoarseness whereas complete voice loss and severe narrowing of the airway occurs when the nerves of both sides are injured.

The external branch of the superior laryngeal nerve passes alongside the superior thyroid arteries to supply the cricothyroid muscle. In thyroidectomy the nerve may be damaged when ligating these vessels. Damage to the external branch of the superior laryngeal nerve eliminates the tension that the cricothyroid muscle exerts on the vocal cords and results in weakness of phonation and impaired alteration of pitch.

The surgeon is careful to preserve the parathyroid glands.

Q 13. How many parathyroid glands are there and why are they at risk? *2 marks*

A There are two parathyroid glands on each side (1 mark). They are usually embedded in the posterior part (½ mark) of the lobe (½ mark) of the thyroid gland and thus can be inadvertently excised at thyroidectomy.

Q 14. What is the effect of a fall in parathyroid hormone levels (a) on blood calcium and (b) on bone? *2 marks*

A Reduced parathyroid hormone causes reduced serum calcium levels (1 mark) but this has little effect on bone (1 mark).

📁 **LEARNING POINT**

Low serum calcium may lead to tremor, tetany and convulsions.

Miss Taylor was successfully treated with partial thyroidectomy and has experienced no recurrence in her disease. She is concentrating better on her studies and is currently working towards her final exams. However, she is occasionally anxious that her symptoms may return since there is a 5% risk of relapse following surgery.

📖 **BIBLIOGRAPHY**

Ellis H, Calne R, Watson C. 2006. *Lecture Notes. General Surgery*, 11th edn. London: Blackwell Publishing.

Franklyn J A. 1993. Hyperthyroidism. *Med Int*, **21**, 164–169.

Ganong W F. 2005. *Review of Medical Physiology*, 22nd edn. New York: McGraw-Hill Medical.

Kumar P, Clark M. 2005. *Clinical Medicine*, 6th edn. Edinburgh: Elsevier Saunders.

Tortora G J, Grabowski S R. 2000. *Principles of Anatomy and Physiology*, 9th edn. New York: John Wiley and Sons.

ENDOCRINOLOGY

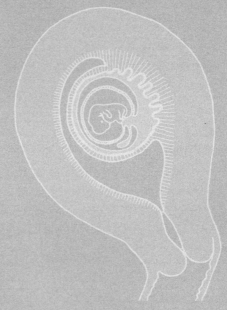

REPRODUCTION CASES: ANSWERS

REPRODUCTION
1. FERTILITY

You are a GP registrar in the middle of a general surgery one afternoon. Your next appointment is for a Mrs Young whom you have not met before. You have a quick look through her medical notes before calling her through. You note that she has a repeat prescription for the combined oral contraceptive pill.

Q **1. What is a 'combined oral contraceptive pill'?** *1 mark*

A The combined oral contraceptive pill consists of oestrogen (½ mark) and a progestogen (½ mark) in varying proportions.

Q **2. Describe the three major actions of the combined oral contraceptive pill.** *3 marks*

A It has three main actions:

o Prevents ovulation – both oestrogen and progestogen inhibit gonadotrophin release from the anterior pituitary (1 mark).

o Inhibits sperm penetration of the cervical mucus – progestogen alters the consistency of the cervical mucus, making it impenetrable to spermatozoa (1 mark)

o Prevents implantation – oestrogen and progestogen result in inadequate endometrial proliferation (1 mark).

Mrs Young has not requested her oral contraceptive prescription for a number of months. You wonder if she is here about a pregnancy.

Q **3. Describe the sequence of events that occur in the ovary during the menstrual cycle under the following headings.** *5 marks*

- Follicular phase (3 marks)

o A groups of follicles in the ovaries are stimulated to develop (½ mark) under the influence of follicle-stimulating hormone (FSH) (½ mark).

o One of the follicles starts to grow rapidly and becomes the dominant (Graafian[a]) follicle (½ mark). As this follicle develops it secretes increasing amounts of oestrogen (½ mark).

o High levels of oestrogen feed back positively (½ mark) to the anterior pituitary to stimulate continued release of follicle-stimulating hormone and luteinising hormone (LH) (½ mark).

- Ovulation (1 mark)

o 14 days before menstruation a surge of LH (½ mark) triggers rupture of the dominant (Graafian) follicle and release of the secondary oocyte (½ mark).

- Luteal phase (1 mark)

o The remaining granulosa cells and theca (½ mark) collapse to form the corpus luteum, which secretes predominantly progesterone and some oestrogen (½ mark).

📁 LEARNING POINT

The surge of LH initiates a final increase in the number of granulosa cells surrounding the primary oocyte and consequently an increase in the secretion of follicular fluid in the Graafian follicle.

It is thought that prostaglandins E_2 and F_2 in the fluid cause the production of proteolytic enzymes, which break down the wall of the Graafian follicle resulting in ovulation.

As soon as the dominant follicle is mature, the primary oocyte completes its meiotic division giving the secondary oocyte and the first polar body. The second maturation division is completed only if the oocyte is fertilised.

REPRODUCTION

Q **4. The following terms describe features of the ovarian follicles. Define each of the terms.** *3 marks*

4(a). Follicular atresia (1 mark).

A The phenomenon that most follicles do not fully mature but degenerate.

4(b). Secondary follicle (1 mark).

A A follicle in which the antrum (fluid-filled cavity) has formed.

4(c). Zona pellucida (1 mark).

A Glycoprotein coat that forms around the oocyte as follicles mature.

Q **5. During a normal menstrual cycle, through which three phases does the endometrium pass and on which days of the cycle do they occur?** *3 marks*

Endometrial phase	Days of menstrual cycle
Menstrual phase	Days 1–3/5
Proliferative phase	Day 3/5–14
Secretory phase	Day 14–28

A 1 mark for being able to name each phase and the corresponding days of the cycle; 3 marks in total.

Mrs Young comes into your surgery looking anxious. Her news is not what you expect. She tells you that she and her husband have been trying unsuccessfully to conceive for the last six months. She is particularly concerned about her husband's fertility as he suffered from mumps when he was 17.

Q **6. What is mumps and what organs does it affect?** *3 marks*

A Mumps is a viral infection (1 mark) or mumps is caused by a paramyxovirus (1 mark). It particularly affects the salivary glands (1 mark) and testes (1 mark).

Q 7. Identify A–J on the following diagram (Figure 8.1) of the male reproductive tract. *5 marks*

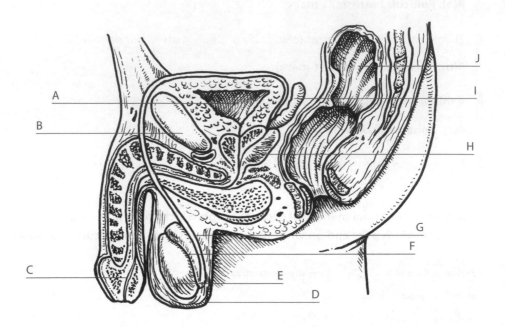

Figure 8.1: The male reproductive tract.

A ½ mark for each of the following:

A – Urinary bladder

B – Pubic symphysis

C – Urethra

D – Scrotum

E – Testis

F – Epididymis

G – Ductus (vas) deferens

H – Prostate

I – Seminal vesicle

J – Rectum

Q **8. At the testis, what is the difference between the tunica vaginalis and the tunica albuginea?** *2 marks*

A The tunica albuginea is the connective tissue capsule of the testis (1 mark).

A The tunica vaginalis is the serous membrane that invests the testis (1 mark).

Q **9. What two cell populations are found in the seminiferous tubules of the testes?** *1 mark*

A Spermatogenic cells and Sertoli[b] cells.

Q **10. Place the following in order of development.** *1 mark*

- **Spermatocyte**
- **Spermatogonium**
- **Spermatid**
- **Spermatozoon**

A Spermatogonium – spermatocyte – spermatid – spermatozoon (1 mark: all four must be in correct order).

Q **11. At which of the above stages is the chromosome number halved by meiosis?** *1 mark*

A Spermatocytes undergo meiosis.

Q **12. What is the function of the interstitial (Leydig[c]) cells of the testes and what controls their function?** *1 mark*

A Testicular interstitial cells secrete testosterone (½ mark) under the influence of luteinising hormone (½ mark) from the anterior pituitary.

LEARNING POINT

Follicle-stimulating hormone (FSH) from the anterior pituitary acts directly on the spermatogonia to stimulate spermatogenesis.

Sertoli cells secrete androgen-binding protein under the influence of FSH and testosterone.

Androgen-binding protein binds to testosterone and keeps its concentration high in the seminiferous tubules.

Testosterone stimulates the final steps of spermatogenesis.

Mrs Young asks how to go about having her husband's fertility checked and wonders about a semen sample.

Q 13. What term is used when there are fewer than 10 million spermatozoa per millilitre? *1 mark*

A Oligospermia.

You explain to Mrs Young that male infertility is a rare complication of mumps but that you would be happy to see her husband to allay any concerns. You advise, however, that fertility tests are stressful and that the majority of patients conceive within a year of regular unprotected sexual intercourse. Mrs Young decides to wait until this time before commencing investigations.

📖 BIBLIOGRAPHY

Fawcett D W. 1994. *A Textbook of Histology*. New York: Chapman and Hall.

Glasier A, Gebbie A. 2000. *Handbook of Family Planning and Reproductive Healthcare*, 4th edn. London: Churchill Livingstone.

Monga A, Campbell S. 2006. *Gynaecology by Ten Teachers*, 18th edn. London: Hodder Arnold.

Sadler T W. 2006. *Langman's Essential Medical Embryology*, 10th edn. London: Lippincott, Williams and Wilkins.

Tortora G J, Grabowski S R. *Principles of Anatomy and Physiology*, 10th edn. New York: John Wiley & Sons.

[a]Regnier de Graaf (1641–1673), Dutch physician and anatomist. Although named after him, the mature or Graafian follicles had been described previously. He was, however, probably the first to appreciate the function of the uterine tubes. De Graaf studied in Delft and Leiden and also in Angers and Paris. Because he was a Catholic in a Protestant country he was unable to follow a university career.

[b]Enrico Sertoli (1842–1910), Italian physiologist and histologist. He described the sustentacular cells of Sertoli in 1865. He later became Professor of Physiology at Milan.

[c]Franz von Leydig (1821–1908), German zoologist and comparative anatomist who discovered the interstitial cells of the testis in 1850. He also defined cell types in the epidermis of fish and amphibians and in connective tissue and blood vessels of crustaceans.

REPRODUCTION
2. PREGNANCY

Two months after her first consultation Mrs Young is once again (see Case 1, Fertility) one of the patients in your afternoon general surgery. This time she looks much happier. She tells you that she thinks she is pregnant as her period is three weeks late and she has had a positive result on a home pregnancy test.

Q 1. Explain how the ELISA (enzyme-linked immunosorbent assay) home pregnancy test works. *2 marks*

- It contains free monoclonal antibody to human chorionic gonadotropin (hCG), coupled to an enzyme (½ mark).

- A second polyclonal antibody to hCG is fixed in the test window and coupled to a substrate dye (½ mark).

- hCG in a pregnant woman's urine binds to the fixed antibody and free antibodies bringing the enzyme and substrate dye into contact thus producing a colour change in the test window (½ mark).

- The test also contains a control window with antibodies as above to human albumin (½ mark).

Q 2. When is human chorionic gonadotropin first detectable in the pregnant woman's urine? *1 mark*

A Immediately after implantation or 6–12 days after fertilisation, or about the first day that the missed menstrual period would have been expected.

Q 3. In the first three months of pregnancy, which tissue produces human chorionic gonadotropin? *1 mark*

A Syncytiotrophoblast.

Q 4. What is the action of human chorionic gonadotropin on the ovary? *1 mark*

A Prevents disintegration of the corpus luteum.

Q 5. In the second and third trimesters, what is the main source of progesterone? *1 mark*

A The placenta.

Q 6. Name two actions of progesterone during pregnancy. *1 mark*

A Any of the following (½ mark each):

- Prevents endometrial shedding
- Prevents myometrial contractions by inhibiting secretion of prostaglandins in the myometrium
- Suppresses ovulation
- Stimulates breast development
- Stimulates appetite and promotes storage of body fat
- Stimulates respiration by sensitising the respiratory centre to CO_2.

Having confirmed Mrs Young's pregnancy you offer her your congratulations as she is obviously very pleased. You ask her the date of the first day of her last period and confirm that she has a regular 28-day menstrual cycle. From this information you estimate that she is about 5 weeks pregnant.

Q 7. Identify A–F on this diagram of the early pregnant uterus (Figure 8.2).   *6 marks*

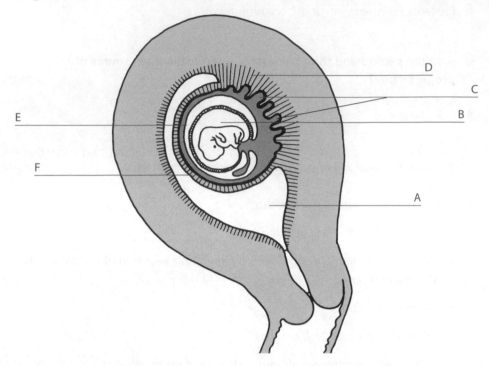

Figure 8.2: The early pregnant uterus.

A 1 mark for each of the following:

A – Uterine cavity

B – Amnionic cavity

C – Placenta (specifically chorion frondosum)

D – Decidua basalis

E – Chorionic cavity

F – Decidua capsularis

Q 8. When does the pregnant uterus first become palpable?   *1 mark*

A At 12 weeks' gestation the pregnant uterus is palpable suprapubically.

Q 9. Name the tissues found in a placental villus at 3 months of pregnancy. *2 marks*

- Syncytiotrophoblast (½ mark).

- Cytotrophoblast (½ mark).

- Extra-embryonic mesoderm (½ mark).

- Fetal capillary endothelium (½ mark).

Q 10. Which tissues form the placental barrier at its thinnest part from the 4th month of pregnancy onwards? *1 mark*

- Syncytiotrophoblast (½ mark).

- Fetal capillary endothelium (½ mark).

Q 11. What is meant by the term 'syncytial knot'? *1 mark*

A Pieces of syncytial trophoblast that break off into the maternal blood.

 LEARNING POINT

Syncytial knots travel to the mother's lungs and degenerate without causing symptoms. Their significance is unknown.

Q 12. Define the following terms. *3 marks*

12(a). Placental cotyledon.

12(b). Placenta praevia.

12(c). Battledore placenta.

A (a) Placental cotyledon: unit of placental structure (1 mark).

A (b) Placenta praevia: placenta covering the internal os (1 mark).

A (c) Battledore placenta: umbilical cord attaching at one side of placenta (1 mark).

REPRODUCTION

LEARNING POINT

Placental cotyledons can break off and be retained at delivery.

Placenta praevia is an important cause of antepartum haemorrhage.

Battledore is another name for a badminton racket. When the umbilical cord is attached at the side of the placenta rather than at its centre, the cord and placenta resemble a badminton racket!

You establish that Mrs Young is still taking the folic acid you advised before conception and reiterate the importance of continuing with this supplement for the first three months of pregnancy to help prevent neural tube defects.

Q 13. What are the three embryonic germ layers? *1½ marks*

- Ectoderm (½ mark).

- Mesoderm (½ mark).

- Endoderm (½ mark).

Q 14. Describe the four major stages in the formation of the neural tube. *2 marks*

- Transformation of the embryonic ectoderm into a thickened neural plate (½ mark).

- Lateral folding of the neural plate (½ mark) along the midline neural groove.

- Apposition and fusion of the neural folds and separation from the overlying ectoderm (½ mark). Closure begins midway along the craniocaudal axis of the neural tube and extends in both directions.

- Closure of the anterior and posterior neuropores (½ mark). This normally occurs during the fourth week.

REPRODUCTION

Q 15. Explain the importance of folate in the prevention of neural tube defects. *1½ marks*

- Folate functions as a single carbon donor (½ mark) in many of the body's metabolic reactions, including the formation of some amino acids, thymidine monophosphate and purine synthesis.

- As such folate is important for protein and DNA synthesis (½ mark).

- The formation of the neural tube is a period of rapid cell proliferation (½ mark) and it is therefore necessary to ensure an adequate dietary intake of folate during this period.

You measure Mrs Young's blood pressure and note that it is relatively low at 102/64 mmHg. You explain that women often have a drop in blood pressure during the first few months of pregnancy.

Q 16. Give two other ways in which the maternal cardiovascular system adapts to pregnancy. *2 marks*

A Any of following (1 mark each):

- Increased heart rate and increased stroke volume resulting in

- Increased cardiac output by 30%–40%

- Increased plasma volume

📁 LEARNING POINT

The fall in systemic vascular resistance is associated with expansion of the placental and renal vasculature and also cutaneous vasodilatation.

The balance between vasoconstriction and vasodilatation in pregnancy is the critical determinant of blood pressure and central to the pathogenesis of pre-eclampsia.

REPRODUCTION

You see from Mrs Young's medical notes that she is blood group O Rhesus negative. You explain to Mrs Young the significance of this for her pregnancy and ask if she knows whether her husband is Rhesus negative or positive. Mrs Young agrees to find out.

Q **17. Explain the significance of a Rhesus negative blood group in a first pregnancy.**

2 marks

A Any four of the following:

- The Rhesus antigen is a red blood cell antigen (½ mark).

- As Mrs Young is Rhesus negative she does not have the antigen on her red cells (½ mark).

- If she is exposed to the antigen from a Rhesus-positive baby at delivery she will form Rhesus antibodies (½ mark).

- In a subsequent pregnancy, these antibodies can cross the placenta (½ mark) and attack the erythrocytes of a Rhesus-positive fetus, causing haemolytic anaemia in utero (½ mark).

📖 **BIBLIOGRAPHY**

Baker P N. 2006. *Obstetrics by Ten Teachers*, 18th edn. London: Hodder Arnold.

Sadler T W. 2006. *Langman's Essential Medical Embryology*, 10th edn. London: Lippincott, Williams and Wilkins.

Standring S. 2005. *Gray's Anatomy*, 39th edn. Edinburgh: Elsevier Churchill Livingstone.

REPRODUCTION

REPRODUCTION
3. PROSTATE

You are the registrar at the urology clinic. One of the patients is Mr Grierson who has been referred by his GP. Mr Grierson is 61 years old. He had been asked to attend the well-man clinic at his GP's surgery and made up his mind it was the opportunity to see the doctor about his prostate problems. His 66-year-old brother, Robert, is being treated for cancer of the prostate and in recent months Mr Grierson has been having to get up through the night to pass urine. He has also been noticing that on voiding urine it is difficult to get the stream started. Mr Grierson has been otherwise well but knows that these are signs of prostatic disease but had been putting off seeking help.

Q **1. Label the following on the diagram (Figure 8.3):**

- **Anal canal**
- **Bulb of penis**
- **Bulbospongiosus muscle**
- **Corpus cavernosum**
- **Corpus spongiosum**
- **Ductus (vas) deferens**
- **Ejaculatory duct**
- **Neck of bladder**
- **Prostate**
- **Urethral sphincter**

A (½ mark for each, 5 marks in total)

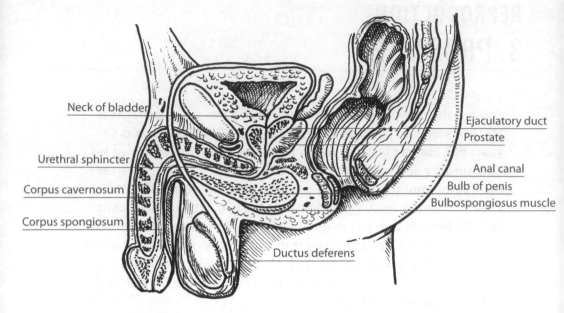

Figure 8.3: Male reproductive tract.

The sensation of needing to pass urine comes from stretch receptors in the wall of the urinary bladder as it comes under tension.

Q 2. To which segments of the spinal cord do primary sensory neuron pass from the bladder? *1 mark*

A T10–L2 (½ mark) and S2–S4 (½ mark).

📁 LEARNING POINT

These are the same segments from which the sympathetic and parasympathetic supplies, respectively, to the bladder arise.

Having listened to the history you take a blood sample for analysis of urea and electrolytes and for prostate-specific antigen.

Q 3. What is prostate-specific antigen? *1 mark*

A Prostate-specific antigen is a protein (1 mark) produced by the prostatic epithelial cells.

Q 4. Give four situations in which serum levels of prostate-specific antigen are likely to be raised. *2 marks*

- Prostatic cancer (½ mark).
- Prostatic hypertrophy (½ mark).
- Recent ejaculation (½ mark).
- Prostatitis (½ mark).

 LEARNING POINT

It is a myth that digital rectal examination raises levels of prostate-specific antigen (Kumar and Clark 2005).

You carry out a rectal examination to check for prostatic hypertrophy or prostatic cancer.

Q 5. How would you distinguish these two conditions at rectal examination? *2 mark*

A In cancer of the prostate, enlargement is irregular (½ mark) in contour and heterogeneous (½ mark) in texture. In benign prostatic hyperplasia, enlargement is diffuse (½ mark) and firm and smooth (½ mark) in texture.

Q 6. What is the rectovesical pouch and is it palpable at rectal examination? *3 marks*

A The rectovesical pouch is the most inferior part (1 mark) of the peritoneum in the male subject (1 mark). It is too far from the anal margin to be palpable at rectal examination (1 mark). In the female, however, the rectouterine pouch is more inferiorly placed and can be reached by the examining finger.

REPRODUCTION

At rectal examination, you palpate a symmetrical diffuse enlargement of rubbery consistency. A longitudinal groove is palpable in the midline and the rectal mucosa moves freely relative to the prostate.

Q **7. Are these abnormal features?** *2 marks*

A The diffuse enlargement is abnormal (½ mark).

A The rubbery consistency (½ mark), the longitudinal groove (½ mark) and the mobile rectal mucosa (½ mark) are all normal features.

Q **8. Why are urea and electrolytes checked?** *1 mark*

A Prostatic enlargement can impair urinary flow and lead to renal failure.

The urea and electrolytes prove to be in the normal range and the prostate-specific antigen levels show borderline elevation. The diagnosis is benign prostatic hypertrophy.

Q **9. Does the fact that Mr Grierson's brother has prostatic cancer increase his risk of developing the disease?** *1 mark*

A Yes.

 LEARNING POINT

In general the risk of developing prostate cancer is doubled if a man's father or brother has had the disease.

Arrangements are made for Mr Grierson to have a transurethral resection of his prostate. He is a very well-informed man with a sharp mind and wants to know about the procedure and the possible risks of the surgery, especially with regard to urinary continence and sexual function.

Q 10. From the bladder outwards, what are the parts of the male urethra and what are the approximate lengths of each part? *3 marks*

Prostatic part: 3–4 cm (1 mark).

Membranous part: 1–2 cm (1 mark).

Spongiose (penile) part: 15 cm (1 mark).

A (Must get both the name and the length of part for each mark.)

Q 11. The urethral (external) sphincter is the main muscle controlling continence of urine. Which part of the urethra does it surround? What is its nerve supply? *2 marks*

A It surrounds the membranous urethra (1 mark). It is supplied by the pudendal nerve (1 mark).

📁 LEARNING POINT

The urethral sphincter is composed of skeletal muscle and is under voluntary control.

Q 12. Which muscle helps expel the last drops of urine? *1 mark*

A Bulbospongiosus muscle.

REPRODUCTION

519

Q 13. Which nerves innervate the blood vessels of the corpora cavernosa or spongiosum and are responsible for initiating erection? *1 mark*

A Pelvic splanchnic nerves (1 mark) or nervi erigentes (1 mark) or parasympathetic nerves (1 mark).

Q 14. In a healthy subject what prevents the ejaculate from entering the urinary bladder? *1 mark*

A The vesical (internal) sphincter.

📁 LEARNING POINT

While the above is believed to be true, the details of the structure and function of the vesical sphincter around the urethra as it leaves the bladder are controversial and incompletely understood.

The transurethral resection of the prostate is carried out under general anaesthetic. Samples of prostatic tissue are sent for pathology to exclude carcinoma.

Q 15. Briefly describe the appearance of prostate tissue on light microscopy. *1 mark*

A Glandular tissue with simple columnar epithelium (½ mark) embedded in a fibromuscular (½ mark) stroma.

Q 16. What are amyloid bodies? *1 mark*

A Amyloid bodies (corpora amylacea or prostatic concretions) are eosinophilic bodies in the lumens (1 mark) of the prostatic glands.

Q 17. What type of nerve fibre innervates the smooth muscle of the prostate that contracts at ejaculation?   *1 mark*

A Sympathetic.

In the first two days after surgery, Mr Grierson is alarmed by the presence of blood clots in his urine.

Q 18. What is the likely source of these blood clots?   *1 mark*

A The venous plexus deep to the capsule of the prostate.

📖 BIBLIOGRAPHY

http://www.cancer.org/docroot/CRI/content/CRI_2_4_3X_Can_prostate_cancer_be_found_early_36.asp

Browse N L. 1991. *An Introduction to the Symptoms and Signs of Surgical Disease*, 2nd edn. London: Edward Arnold.

Kumar P, Clark M. 2005. *Clinical Medicine*, 6th edn. Edinburgh: Elsevier Saunders.

Sinnatamby C S. 1999. *Last's Anatomy: Regional and Applied*, 10th edn. Edinburgh: Churchill Livingstone.

Standring S. 2005. *Gray's Anatomy*, 39th edn. Edinburgh: Elsevier Churchill Livingstone.

Steinberg G D, Carter B S, Beaty T H, Childs B, Walsh P C. 1990. Family history and the risk of prostate cancer. *Prostate*, **17**, 337–47.

Tortora G J, Grabowski S R. *Principles of Anatomy and Physiology*, 10th edn. New York: John Wiley & Sons.

REPRODUCTION

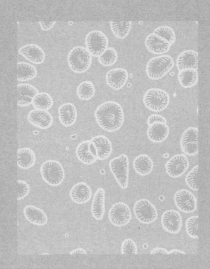

HAEMATOLOGY CASES: ANSWERS

HAEMATOLOGY
1. CHRONIC LYMPHOCYTIC LEUKAEMIA

You are a GP registrar called to the local residential home to assess Mr Burns, a 79-year-old man who has not been feeling well of late. His daughter has become increasingly worried about her father's well being. He is tired and breathless and has multiple unexplained bruises, particularly on his lower limbs.

On examination you discover he has hepatosplenomegaly and has evidence of bleeding into his oral mucosa.

Q 1. In a healthy adult, in which region of the abdominal cavity does the spleen normally lie? *1 mark*

A The left hypochondrium.

Q 2. At the level of which ribs does the spleen lie? *1 mark*

A Level of left 9th to 11th ribs.

Q 3. List four structures that lie between the spleen and the lower left ribs. *2 marks*

A The peritoneum (½ mark).

The diaphragm (½ mark).

The left lung (½ mark).

The pleural cavity or the pleura (½ mark).

HAEMATOLOGY

Q 4. Through which fold of peritoneum does the splenic artery pass to reach the spleen?

1 mark

A Lienorenal ligament.

Q 5. On the following CT of the upper abdomen (Figure 9.1), identify A–J.

5 marks

A ½ mark for each of the following:

A – Rectus abdominis muscle

B – Left lobe of liver

C – Inferior vena cava

D – Diaphragm

E – Splenic flexure of colon

F – Stomach

G – Splenic artery

H – Left kidney

I – Spinal cord

J – Erector spinae muscle

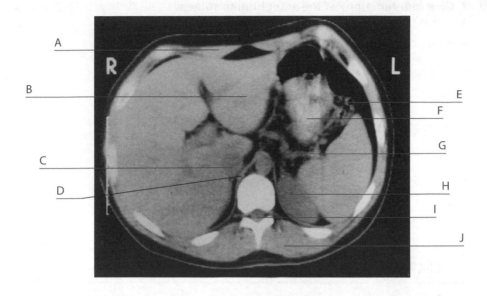

Figure 9.1: CT of the upper abdomen.

The spleen is composed of red pulp and white pulp.

Q **6. Complete the table below indicating whether the features listed belong to the red or white pulp.** *3 marks*

A ½ mark for each correct answer

Feature	Red pulp or white pulp?
Aggregates of lymphocytes	White
Splenic cords	Red
Splenic sinusoids	Red
Central arterioles	White
Lymphoid nodules	White
Penicillar arteries	Red

Q 7. **Give four functions of the adult human spleen.**   *2 marks*

A Any four of the following (½ mark for each):

- Storage of iron.

- Phagocytosis of old/damaged erythrocytes.

- Phagocytosis of old/damaged white blood cells.

- Immune response to circulating antigens.

- Production of B cells and T cells.

A Not enough to say filtration of the blood.

 LEARNING POINT

The spleen is the organ that is most commonly damaged in abdominal trauma. Severe blows over the lower left chest area or upper abdomen can fracture the ribs overlying the spleen and can cause it to rupture. This causes significant haemorrhage and perhaps shock. Immediate removal of the spleen (splenectomy) is likely to be required to prevent death from bleeding. A person can live without the spleen as other structures, such as the red bone marrow and liver, take over some of the functions carried out by the spleen. A splenectomised patient has reduced immunity to infection and prophylactic antibiotics and vaccinations are advised, particularly against pneumococcal and other infections involving encapsulated bacteria. Nowadays attempts are therefore made to preserve the traumatised spleen. Instead of routine splenectomy the spleen can be enclosed and compressed to control bleeding and allow repair.

Mr Burns is found to be anaemic, with a high white cell count, and his platelets are extremely low (thrombocytopaenia). Differential white cell count shows a lymphocytosis.

The haematologist takes charge of Mr Burns's management and admits him to hospital for further investigations. She carries out a bone marrow trephine and aspirate.

Q 8. From which anatomical site are these samples most likely to be taken? *1 mark*

A Iliac crest.

Q 9. For what purpose is: (a) a trephine sample and (b) an aspirate sample collected? *2 marks*

A A trephine allows the overall architecture of the tissue sample to be studied (1 mark).

A An aspirate allows better visualisation of individual cells (1 mark).

A diagnosis of chronic lymphocytic leukaemia is made and Mr Burns is transferred to a side room, as he is vulnerable to infection.

Q 10. Explain why Mr Burns is vulnerable to infection. *1 mark*

A Normal haemopoiesis has been crowded out by production of neoplastic lymphocytes (½ mark).

A Deficiency of normal leukocyte production leads to failure to control infection (½ mark).

Q 11. Why is he anaemic and thrombocytopaenic? *1 mark*

A Again this is due to infiltration of marrow by neoplastic cells to the detriment of normal haematopoiesis.

Q 12. Which cell type is responsible for the production of platelets? *1 mark*

A Megakaryocytes.

Q 13. Complete this flow diagram (Figure 9.2) showing the different cell lines that occur in haemopoiesis. *4 marks*

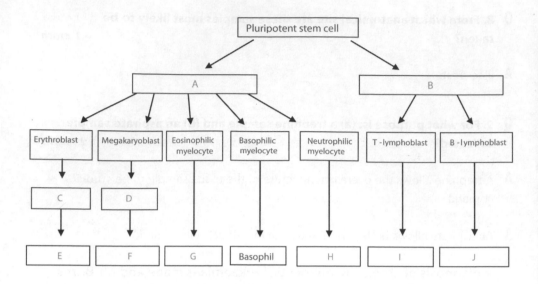

Figure 9.2: Haemopoiesis.

A 1/3 mark for each:

A – Myeloid stem cell

B – Lymphoid stem cell

C – Reticulocyte or normoblast

D – Megakaryocyte

E – Erythrocyte

F – Platelets

G – Eosinophil

H – Neutrophil

I – T-lymphocyte

J – B-lymphocyte

On the ward, Mr Burns requires a special form of nursing known as 'reverse barrier nursing'.

Q 14. What is meant by this term? *1 mark*

A Reverse barrier nursing is when a patient is kept isolated (½ mark) not because they are infectious but because they are particularly vulnerable to infection (½ mark).

Q 15. Give two examples of precautions that would be taken when entering the patient's room. *2 marks*

A Any two of the following (1 mark each):

- Sterilise equipment before coming into contact with the patient, eg cutlery.

- Staff and visitors should wear protective clothing to prevent their microbiological flora from contaminating the patient.

- Adequate hand washing is required, particularly when hospital personnel move from patient to patient.

- None of the equipment used to examine or treat the patient should be used elsewhere, eg personal stethoscope.

As part of his treatment, Mr Burns requires a blood transfusion.

Blood used for transfusion is collected from donors and is processed into different blood components and products.

Q 16. Name two blood components and two blood products. *2 marks*

A Any two from each category (½ mark each):

A Blood components:

- Red cell concentrates

- Platelet concentrates

- Granulocyte concentrates

- Fresh frozen plasma

HAEMATOLOGY

A Blood products:

- Coagulation factor concentrates
- Albumin
- Immunoglobulin
- Cryoprecipitate

📖 BIBLIOGRAPHY

Abrahams P, Craven J, Lumley J. 2005. *Illustrated Clinical Anatomy*. London: Hodder Arnold.

Kumar P, Clark M. 2005. *Clinical Medicine*, 6th edn. Edinburgh: Elsevier Saunders.

Provan D, Krentz A. 2002. *Oxford Handbook of Clinical and Laboratory Investigation*. Oxford: Oxford University Press.

Sanders S, Dawson J, Datta S, Eccles S. 2005. *Oxford Handbook for the Foundation Programme*. Oxford: Oxford University Press.

Stevens A, Lowe J S. 2005. *Human Histology*, 3rd edn. Philadelphia: Elsevier Mosby.

Tortora G J, Derrickson B. 2006. *Principles of Anatomy and Physiology*, 11th edn. Hoboken, New Jersey: Wiley.

HAEMATOLOGY

HAEMATOLOGY
2. IRON DEFICIENCY ANAEMIA

You are a final year medical student attached to a general practice. A 42-year-old woman, Mrs Forbes, comes to the surgery because she becomes tired easily when doing any physical work, even of a minor nature. The GP asks you to take a history from the patient. After asking a series of questions, you are surprised to find the patient has had heavy periods for the past year but has never sought medical help. You suspect iron deficiency anaemia due to chronic blood loss from menorrhagia. On examination Mrs Forbes has angular stomatitis and a smooth tongue.

Q 1. Define the term anaemia. *1 mark*

A Reduction in haemoglobin concentration (½ mark) below the normal range for an age-/sex-matched population (½ mark).

You remember the production of red blood cells (erythropoiesis) requires certain essential micronutrients and hormonal factors.

Q 2. Name two micronutrients, apart from iron, that are essential in erythropoiesis. *2 marks*

A Any two of the following:

- Folate (1 mark).

- Vitamin B$_{12}$ (1 mark).

- Vitamin B$_6$ (1 mark).

You know that erythropoietin (EPO) is the principal hormone regulating the process of erythropoiesis.

Q 3. What is the major site of production in a healthy adult?   *1 mark*

A Peritubular interstitial cells of the kidney (1 mark).

The kidney (½ mark).

Q 4. What is the major stimulus for its production?   *1 mark*

A Hypoxia.

Red cell production and maturation take place in bone marrow and peripheral blood.

Q 5. The flow chart below (Figure 9.3) shows the process of erythropoiesis. Name A, B and C.   *3 marks*

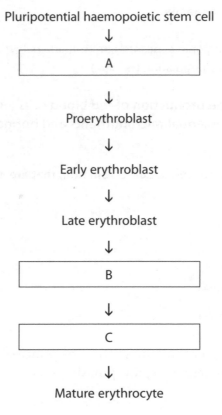

Figure 9.3: Erythropoiesis.

HAEMATOLOGY

A – Myeloid stem cell

B – Normoblast

C – Reticulocyte

Q **6. Name the erythrocyte precursor cell in which each of the following events/features are observed:**

Q **6(a). Extrusion of the nucleus.** *1 mark*

A Normoblast/orthochromic erythroblast.

Q **6(b). The last erythrocyte precursor to contain ribosomes that, on staining for light microscopy, give a blue tinge to the cytoplasm.** *1 mark*

A Reticulocyte.

Q **6(c). The erythrocyte precursor that may appear in increased numbers in the peripheral blood following blood loss.** *1 mark*

A Reticulocyte.

📁 **LEARNING POINT**

Regulation of erythropoiesis

A feedback loop involving erythropoietin helps regulate the process of erythropoiesis so that, in non-disease states, the production of red blood cells is equal to the destruction of red blood cells and the red blood cell number is sufficient to sustain adequate tissue oxygen levels. In the adult 85% of erythropoietin production, as judged by the presence of messenger RNA, takes place in the kidney with 15% in the liver. Increased production occurs primarily in response to low oxygen levels, although androgens, catecholamines and alkalosis also favour increased release. In addition, erythropoietin is bound by circulating red blood cells. Low circulating numbers of erythrocytes leads to a relatively high level of unbound erythropoietin, which stimulates production in the bone marrow.

HAEMATOLOGY

The GP takes a blood sample from Mrs Forbes for full blood count and iron status, the working diagnosis being iron deficiency anaemia due to menorrhagia. While awaiting the result the GP asks you what you expect the results of the blood test will be if this is correct.

Q 7. Fill in the table below, indicating the expected results as increased, decreased or normal.   *3 marks*

Parameter	Result
Haemoglobin	Decreased
Mean cell volume (MCV)	Decreased
Mean cell haemoglobin concentration (MCHC)	Decreased
Serum iron	Decreased
Total iron binding capacity (TIBC)	Increased
Serum ferritin	Decreased

🗁 LEARNING POINT

Total iron binding capacity (TIBC)

Measurement of iron binding capacity is effectively a functional measurement of transferrin (protein that transports iron) concentration. Increased TIBC may occur in iron deficiency, acute infection, childhood, pregnancy and in patients on oral contraceptives. Decreased TIBC may occur in iron overload, cirrhosis of the liver, chronic inflammatory disease and protein-losing states.

The film below is that of the patient (Figure 9.4).

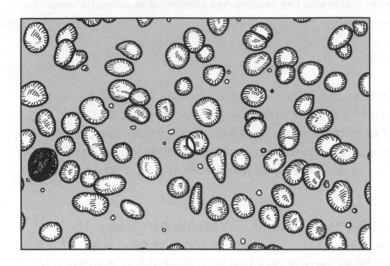

Figure 9.4: Blood film.

Q **8. Give two features of the blood film that indicate iron deficiency anaemia.** *2 marks*

A Microcytic (small erythrocytes) (1 mark).

A Hypochromia (central pallor of erythrocytes) (1 mark).

The white blood cell to the left of the microscope field has a diameter similar to that of healthy erythrocytes.

Q **9. What is this cell?** *1 mark*

A Small (½ mark) lymphocyte (½ mark).

Q **10. Name one other formed element of blood visible in the drawing.** *1 mark*

A Platelets.

Q 11. In patients such as Mrs Forbes with glossitis due to iron deficiency anaemia, what feature of the tongue has atrophied to give the smooth appearance? *1 mark*

A Filiform papillae.

The GP also takes a full gynaecological history from the patient as she has had heavy menstrual periods for the past one year. Abdominal examination reveals a mass arising from the pelvis. Your GP refers the patient to the gynaecological department for further investigation. In the meantime, Mrs Forbes is prescribed ferrous sulphate.

One month later, Mrs Forbes returns to your GP surgery. The iron tablets have been making her constipated. The main reason for her current visit, however, is a problem with swallowing, particularly with solid foods.

Q 12. Label the parts shown in the figure below (Figure 9.5). *6 marks*

A ½ mark for each

A – Sphenoidal sinus

B – Auditory tube

C – Soft palate

D – Body of 3rd cervical vertebra

E – Epiglottis

F – Vocal fold

G – Bony palate

H – Tongue

Figure 9.5: Throat anatomy.

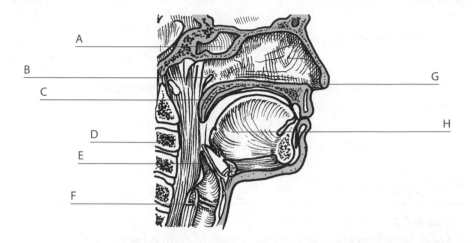

In swallowing, reflexes move the bolus through the pharynx.

Q 13. Which muscle of the tongue moves the tongue backwards and upwards (posterosuperiorly)? *1 mark*

A Styloglossus muscle.

Q 14. Which cranial nerve provides most of the sensory innervation of the oropharynx? *1 mark*

A Glossopharyngeal nerve/CN IX.

Q 15. Indicate which of the following phases of swallowing are voluntary and which are involuntary? *1½ marks*

Phase	Type of movement	Marks
Oral phase	Voluntary	½
Pharyngeal phase	Involuntary	½
Oesophageal phase	Involuntary	½

HAEMATOLOGY

Q 16. Name the principal muscles that move the bolus through the pharynx. ½ *mark*

A Constrictor muscles.

Q 17. What is the main factor preventing food from entering the larynx? *1 mark*

A Sphincter mechanism.

 LEARNING POINT

Oral phase
- Food rolled into bolus and tongue arches to push it backwards

Pharyngeal phase
- Elevation of soft palate (closes nasopharynx)
- Pressure of food on pharyngeal wall stimulates receptors and this activates reflexes which: (a) inhibit respiration, (b) raise the larynx and (c) close the glottis
- Passage of food bolus downwards tilts the epiglottis backwards
- A wave of contractions sweep through the pharyngeal muscles and food is propelled towards the upper oesophageal sphincter

Oesophageal phase
- Reflex relaxation of the upper oesophageal sphincter
- Sphincter closes when food has passed
- Glottis opens and breathing is resumed
- Peristaltic waves propel food forward
- Lower oesophageal sphincter relaxes and food enters the stomach

---

The GP is concerned that Mrs Forbes may have chronic pharyngo-oesophagitis (Paterson–Brown–Kelly[a] disease/Plummer Vinson[b] syndrome), a condition associated with iron deficiency anaemia, and refers her to the ear, nose and throat department for further assessment.

HAEMATOLOGY

The GP sees Mrs Forbes a month later. It had been a uterine fibroid that had been causing the heavy periods. Her problem swallowing is now improving with the iron tablets and she is about to see the otorhinolaryngologist.

📖 BIBLIOGRAPHY

Gray R F, Hawthorne M. 1992. *Synopsis of Otolaryngology*, 5th edn. Oxford: Butterworth Heinemann.

[a]D. R. Paterson (1863–1939) and A. Brown-Kelly (1865–1941), British surgeons who described sideropenic dysphagia independently in 1919.

[b]H. S. Plummer (1874–1936) and P. P. Vinson (1890–1959), American physicians from the Mayo Clinic, Minnesota, who also described the condition in 1912 and 1919 respectively – and whose names are used for its description within the USA.

HAEMATOLOGY

HAEMATOLOGY
3. LYMPH NODES/HIV

You are the GP on duty one afternoon when a 33-year-old patient, Mr Reading, comes to see you because of swellings in his neck and armpits. He has been aware of these for the last four months and has also been feeling tired. He has no previous history of ill health.

After a thorough physical examination, you find that Mr Reading has enlarged lymph nodes, some greater than 2 cm, regular in contour, firm, mobile and non-tender on both sides in his axilla, neck and groin. He also has splenomegaly.

Q **1. List four lymphoid organs or tissues found in humans, apart from lymph nodes.** *2 marks*

A Any four of the following (½ mark each)

- Thymus

- Spleen

- Tonsils

- Mucosa-associated lymphoid tissue and/or Peyer's patches

Most of the lymphoid organs have an internal skeleton of reticular fibres.

Q **2. In brief, what is the composition of reticular fibres?** *1 mark*

A Any one of the following (1 mark):

- Type IV collagen fibres

- Fine collagen fibres

- Fibres that have affinity for silver stains

Q **3. Give two principal functions of a lymph node.**   *2 marks*

A Filtration of lymph (1 mark)

A Immune responses to lymph-borne antigen (1mark)

A diagram of the structure of a lymph node is shown below (Figure 9.6).

Q **4. Identify features A–H (Figure 9.6).**   *4 marks*

Figure 9.6: The structure of a lymph node.

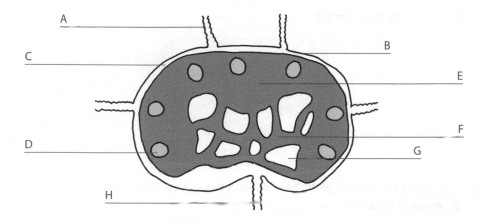

A ½ mark for each:

  A - Afferent lymphatic

  B - Capsule

  C – Subcapsular sinus

  D – Lymphoid nodules (germinal centres)

  E – Deep cortex

  F - Medullary cord

G - Medullary sinus

H - Efferent lymphatic

Q **5. Why are T-lymphocytes called "T"-lymphocytes?** *1 mark*

A The "T" stands for "thymus-dependent" *or* the early cohorts of T-lymphocytes are programmed in the thymus.

Q **6. Which type of lymphocyte, T- or B-, is principally located in the following regions of a lymph node?** *1½ marks*

- **The outer cortex**
- **The deep cortex**
- **The medullary cords?**

A ½ mark for each of the following:

- Outer cortex – B-lymphocytes
- Deep cortex – T-lymphocytes
- Medullary cords – B-lymphocytes

Q **7. Name the immunoglobulin-producing cell type that is derived from B-lymphocytes.** *½ mark*

A Plasma cell.

On looking at his past notes you see that Mr Reading is a recovered heroin addict who was using intravenous drugs for three years before entering a rehabilitation programme. He has now been free of drug abuse for 1 year.

In view of Mr Reading's history you feel that a human immune deficiency virus (HIV) test would be appropriate. He consents to this and admits that the possibility of HIV had been worrying him for some time.

HAEMATOLOGY

Q **8. What type of virus is HIV?** *1 mark*

A ½ mark each for two of these:

HIV is a single-stranded

RNA

Retrovirus

Q **9. Which enzyme is used by viruses such as HIV to form DNA for inclusion in the host genome?** *1 mark*

A Reverse transcriptase.

Q **10. A drawing of this virus is shown below (Figure 9.7). Please name the indicated features.** *2 marks*

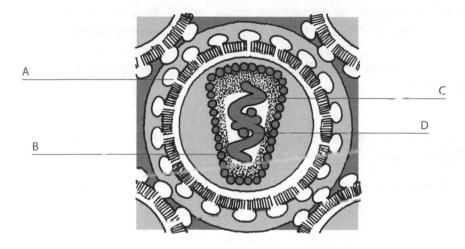

Figure 9.7: The human immunodeficiency virus.

A Features to be labelled (½ mark for each):

A – Glycoprotein

B – Capsid

C – RNA

D – Reverse transcriptase

Q 11. Outline six main steps involved in replication of HIV in vivo.   *3 marks*

A ½ mark for each of the following:

- Attachment and binding to viral receptors on host cells/CD4 receptor

- Fusion of envelope and penetration

- Uncoating

- Transcription of a DNA copy from RNA genome using reverse transcriptase

- Transcription of new viral mRNA in nucleus from DNA

- Production of viral peptide and its release into blood

Q 12. Name the specific cell type which is reduced in HIV infection.   *1 mark*

A $CD4^+$ cells.

(Note macrophages, Langerhans cells and dendritic cells are all invaded at some point – but CD4 cells are the important target. No marks for the others.)

You believe that Mr Reading is probably in the latent period of infection.

Q 13. List the five clinical stages of infection for HIV including the latent period.   *4 marks*

- Incubation (1 mark)

- Seroconversion/asymptomatic (1 mark)

- Latent period/asymptomatic (no marks)

- Symptomatic HIV infection (1 mark)

- Acute immune deficiency syndrome/AIDS/ full-blown AIDS (1 mark)

HAEMATOLOGY

🗁 LEARNING POINT

Incubation

Two to four weeks immediately following infection, usually silent clinically and serologically

Primary infection

- Self-limiting: usually recovery in 1–2 weeks

- Majority are silent

- Symptoms include: fever, sore throat, fatigue, arthralgia, myalgia, mucosal ulcers of mouth and genitals, transient pink maculopapular rash, lymphadenopathy

- Neurological symptoms are common, include headaches, photophobia, myelopathy, neuropathy and rarely encephalopathy

Latent period

- Variable length of time 5–10 years, but up to 15 years is possible

- Clinically well but infectious

- Viral load reaches a set point, balance between rate of viral production and rate of clearance

- Subset of patients have persistent generalised lymphadenopathy: this is what Mr Reading presents with and is classified as nodes > 1 cm diameter at more than two extra-inguinal sites, persisting for 3 months or longer. Nodes are usually bilaterally symmetrical, firm, mobile, non-tender. There may be associated splenomegaly

Symptomatic HIV Infection

- The HIV infection progresses, viral load rises and CD4 count falls

- Patient can develop an array of symptoms and signs. The clinical picture will be a result of direct HIV effects and associated immunosuppression

HAEMATOLOGY

Q 14. Give three modes of transmission of HIV. *1 mark*

A Any three of these for 1 mark:

- Unprotected sex

- Contaminated needles

- Contaminated blood/blood products, eg transplants and blood transfusions

- Mother to child, ie vertical transmission (birth and breast milk)

Mr Reading wishes to know about treatment. Although there is no current treatment to completely eradicate infection, there are drugs that can suppress the virus even below limits of detection. You tell him that anti-retroviral drugs are the main method of treatment.

Q 15. Explain how these drugs work. *2 marks*

A There are three types which act by:

- o Inhibit HIV enzyme reverse transcriptase which allows HIV RNA to be transcribed into DNA and ultimately make a copy of itself (1 mark)

- o Protease inhibitors which act to inhibit HIV protease enzyme, which cleaves viral proteins (1 mark)

Q 16. What tests could you do to monitor Mr Reading's progress? *1 mark*

- CD4 count (½ mark)

- HIV RNA levels (viral load) (½ mark)

Q 17. Give two other pieces of advice you would like to tell Mr Reading. *1 mark*

A Two of the following for 1 mark:

- Explain the regimes of drugs are complex and that strict adherence to regime is necessary

- Need for safe sex at all times

HAEMATOLOGY

- Need to inform partners

- Dietary assessment and advice/referral to dietician

- General health promotion advice on smoking, alcohol, drugs, exercise

Q 18. Finally, name the primary opportunistic infection seen in HIV disease. *1 mark*

A Mycobacterium tuberculosis.

📖 REFERENCES

Boon NA, Colledge NR, Walker BR, Hunter JAA. 2006. *Davidson's Principles and Practice of Medicine*, 20th edn. Edinburgh: Elsevier Churchill Livingstone.

British National Formulary – September 2004. London: British Medical Association, Royal Pharmaceutical Society of Great Britain.

Kumar P, Clark M. 1998. *Clinical Medicine*. London: WB Saunders.

Longmore M, Wilkinson I, Turmezei T, Cheung CK, Smith E. 2007. *Oxford Handbook of Clinical Medicine,* 7th edn. Oxford: Oxford University Press.

Mims C, Dockrell M, Goering R, Roitt I, Wakelin D, Zuckerman M. 2004. *Medical Microbiology*, 3rd edn. London: Mosby.

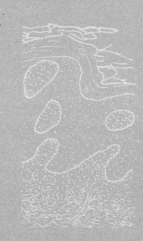

DERMATOLOGY CASE:
ANSWERS

DERMATOLOGY
1. PSORIASIS

You are on duty in general practice one morning. The next patient to arrive is Miss Smith, an anxious 15-year-old girl who has come along to see you with her mother. She is embarrassed, as recently she has noticed skin changes particularly on her arms and around her knees.

On examination, you notice that there are numerous small round red plaques, with obvious scaling, present on her forearms, elbows, knees and shins. You make the diagnosis of psoriasis.

Q 1. What form of psoriasis is this most likely to be?   *1 mark*

A Guttate psoriasis.

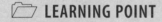 LEARNING POINT

Between 1% and 3% of the population is affected by psoriasis, peak onset being between the ages of 15 and 40, both sexes affected equally. European and North American white people are the most affected, whereas it is less prevalent in North American black people. It is a chronic (with exacerbations and remissions), inflammatory skin condition which is non-infectious. It is characterised by well-defined scaling plaques. The majority of cases are relatively mild and medical attention may not be sought.

Q 2. Describe *four* characteristic histological features of the skin in this disease.   *4 marks*

A Any four of the following:

- Hyperproliferation of keratinocytes, resulting in irregular thickening of the epidermis (½ mark) called acanthosis (for full 1 mark)

DERMATOLOGY

- Parakeratosis, ie nuclei are retained in the stratum corneum/horny layer (1 mark)

- Loss of granular layer (1 mark)

- Dilatation and elongation of capillary loops in the dermal papillae (1 mark)

- Infiltration of the epidermis and dermis by inflammatory cells (neutrophils, macrophages, lymphocytes and dendritic cells) (1 mark)

🗂 LEARNING POINT

The *pathogenesis* of psoriasis is still not entirely understood. It is thought to be an immune-mediated disease, in which lymphocytes release cytokines, resulting in epidermal and capillary proliferation. Growth factors, eg tumour necrosis factor α, interleukins 2 and 8 and interferon γ, are also likely to be involved in acting on the epidermis.

The *aetiology* of psoriasis is multifactorial, with genetic and environmental factors both playing a role:

Genetic

There is a positive family history in ~30% of cases, with high (73%) concordance rates for identical twins. Nine genetic loci (PSORS1–9) have been identified

Environmental

May trigger onset in an individual who is genetically susceptible, or exacerbate existing disease/cause relapse
- *Infection* – in adolescents, streptococcal throat infection can often trigger the guttate form of psoriasis. HIV infection is also implicated
- *Medication* – drugs that exacerbate psoriasis include lithium, antimalarials, non-steroidal anti-inflammatory drugs and beta-blockers
- *Trauma* – can be psychological (eg stress in some patients) or physical
- *Alcohol* – is thought to have an effect in precipitating or maintaining psoriasis
- *Smoking* – high concordance rates in those patients with palmoplantar pustular psoriasis

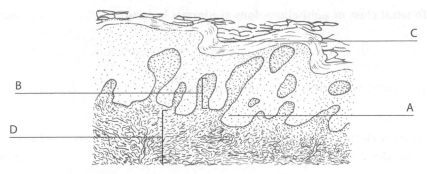

Figure 10.1: Skin structure.

Q 3. Label normal skin structures A–D   *2 marks*

A – Stratum basale (½ mark) or rete ridge (½ mark)

B - Dermal papilla (½ mark)

C – Stratum corneum (½ mark)

D – Dermis (½ mark)

📁 **LEARNING POINT**

The skin is the body's largest organ. Its functions include thermoregulation, gathering sensory information from the environment, playing an active role in the immune system and being a protective barrier.

The *epidermis* is the outer skin layer. It contains no blood vessels and is composed of different layers (strata basale, spinosum, granulosum, lucidum and corneum). Note: stratum lucidum only found in hands and feet, ie thick skin.

The *dermis* forms the bulk of the skin. It provides support to the overlying epidermis, supplying it with nutrients. Collagen and elastin allow the dermis to have strength and yet be flexible. A layer of subcutaneous fat separates the dermis from underlying muscle and fascia.

Q 4. To what class of epithelium does epidermis belong?   *1 mark*

A Stratified squamous (½ mark), keratinised (½ mark) epithelium.

The normal epidermis is 50–150 µm thick.

Q 5. How much thicker can epidermis be in psoriasis, when compared with healthy skin?   *1 mark*

A 3–5× normal.

Keratinocytes are the main type of cell found in skin (~85%). These are held together by different types of intercellular contacts.

Q 6. Complete the table, giving the function of the following intercellular junctions (not specific to skin).   *2 marks*

A Any four of the following, ½ mark each:

Name of junction	Function
Tight junction	Barrier to passage of materials between cells into extracellular space (½ mark)
Gap junction	Gives route for cell-to-cell communication (½ mark), allows metabolite exchange (½ mark) electrical communication (½ mark)
Desmosome	Points of mechanical adherence between cells (½ mark)
Hemidesmosome	Attachment point to underlying basal lamina (½ mark)

Q 17. How do they work? *1 mark*

A Any two of the following:

- They influence vitamin D receptors in keratinocytes (½ mark)

- Inhibit keratinocyte production (½ mark)

- Induce terminal differentiation (½ mark)

- Exert an immunological effect (½ mark)

📁 **LEARNING POINT**

Management

Psoriasis can be managed in a variety of different ways. Lifestyle changes, including the reduction of cigarette smoking and alcohol, can be beneficial in some patients.

Topical treatments are considered the safest, and include emollients, tar, vitamin D analogues, dithranol, corticosteroids and retinoids.

Ultraviolet radiation (UVB) can be used 2–3 times per week for up to 8 weeks. The main risk in the short-term of this form of treatment is acute phototoxicity (sunburn) and in the long term it may increase the risk of skin cancer.

Systemic treatment can be employed if the above therapies fail to work, eg oral retinoids for severe erythrodermic or pustular psoriasis. Low-dose oral methotrexate or cyclosporin also can be effective. Toxicity, however, often limits their long-term use.

PUVA (photochemotherapy) is a form of treatment in which photosensitising agents are taken by mouth, followed by exposure to long-wave ultraviolet radiation (UVA). The main side-effect is painful erythema and one quarter of patients experience itching during and immediately after radiation exposure. It is used less frequently now, as a high cumulative dose significantly increases the risk of skin cancer.

Q 18. Complete this table.   *3 marks*

An example of vitamin D analogue	Advantages of vitamin D analogues (give 2)	Disadvantages of vitamin D analogues (give 2)
Calcipotriol, or Calcitriol, or Tacalcitol (1 mark)	Effective, clean, convenient (½ for each – 1 mark total)	Need constant treatment as remission is short Skin irritation Greasy in nature Small risk of hypercalcaemia if overdose (½ for 2 – 1 mark total)

📖 BIBLIOGRAPHY

Hunter J A A, Savin J A, Dahl M V. 2002. *Clinical Dermatology*, 3rd edn. Oxford: Blackwell Science.

Kumar P, Clark M. 2005. *Clinical Medicine*, 6th edn. Edinburgh: Elsevier Saunders.

Longmore M, Wilkinson I, Turmezei T, Cheung CK, Smith E. 2007. *Oxford Handbook of Clinical Medicine*, 7th edn. Oxford: Oxford University Press.

MacKie R M. 2003. *Clinical Dermatology*, 5th edn. Oxford: Oxford University Press.

McPhee S J, Ganong W F. 2006. *Pathophysiology of Disease*, 5th edn. New York: Lange Medical Books/McGraw-Hill.

[a]Paul Langerhans (see page 483).

[b]Friedrich Sigmund Merkel (1845–1919), German anatomist and histopathologist who described 'Tastzellum' (touch cells) in the skin of vertebrates.

[c]Michael Stanley Clive Birkbeck (1925–2005), British electron microscopist at the Chester Beatty Institute of Cancer Research, London. He discovered the 'tennis-racket' or rod-shaped organelles that are a feature of Langherhans cells.

[d]Heinrich Koebner (1838–1904), German dermatologist. He worked on mycology and sometimes inoculated himself with fungi to demonstate their infectiousness.

[e]Heinrich Auspitz (1835–1886), Austrian dermatologist and tissue pathologist who became professor of dermatology at the University of Vienna.

INDEX

Note: This index covers the answer section only. Page numbers in **bold** indicate the main subject of each case.

splenomegaly 542
statins 349, 442
steatorrhea 360
steroid hormones 480
steroids, oral 337
stomach
   acid secretion 379–80
   epithelial cells 378–9
straight leg raise test 410
stroke 444–5, **462–70**
stroke volume 293
submucous plexus (Meissner's plexus) 353
swallowing 538–40
   difficulties 435
sympathetic nervous system 283, 296
synacthen test 474–5
syncytial knot 511
synovial joints 406
systolic murmur 277–8

taeniae coli 353
testis 505
thiazide diuretics 296, 442
thoracic vertebra, anatomy 459
thoracodorsal nerve 310
throat anatomy 538–9
thrombocytopenia 528
thyroid disease **492–8**
thyroid follicle 493–4
thyroid function tests 496
thyroid gland
   anatomy 495
   enlargement 494
thyroid hormones 492, 494, 496
thyroidectomy, subtotal 497
tongue
   muscles 539
   smooth 532
total iron binding capacity (TIBC) 536
total lung capacity 335
transient ischaemic attack 440, 441
transurethral resection of the prostate 519,

520
trisomy 21 266
trochanteric anastomosis 424
tuberculosis **317–23**

ulcerative colitis 355–6
ulna 407
upper abdomen, anatomy 341–2, 347–8,
   526–7
upper limb
   muscles 401, 406
   peripheral nerves 401–2
   weakness 400–1
upper motor neurone lesion 453
urea and electrolytes analysis
   in diabetes 488
   in prostate disease 516, 518
urethra, male 519
urethral (external) sphincter 519
urine
   continence 519
   darkened 361
   retention 409
   urge to void 516
urobilinogen 346, 361
ursodeoxycholic acid (UDCa) 359
uterus
   fibroids 541
   in pregnancy 510

vagus nerves 283
valvular heart disease 275–82
varicose veins 298
veins, valves 299
venae comitantes 299
venous conditions of the lower limb **298–303**
ventricular performance curve 295
ventricular septal defect (VSD) 259–61, 262,
   268
vertebral canal 413
vesical (internal) sphincter 520

PICTURE PERMISSIONS

The following figures in this book have been reproduced from Tortora and Gradowski (1996, 2002 – 10th e, 2003) Principles of Anatomy and Physiology by kind permission of John Wiley & Sons Inc

Neurology

Figure 6.1 Anatomy of the calf muscles of the right lower limb

Figure 6.3 Attachments of the cranial nerves to the brain

Endocrinology

Figure 7.5 A thyroid follicle

Figure 7.6 Thyroid anatomy

Reproduction

Figures 8.1 & 8.3 The male reproductive tract

The following figure in this book have been reproduced from http://sickle.bwh.harvard.edu/fe-def.html by kind permission of the Division of Haematology, Harvard Medical School, Boston.

Haematology

Figure 9.4 Blood Source

USEFUL WEBSITES

http://www.aic.cuhk.edu.hk/web8

http://www.njsurgery.com/html/anatomy%20lessons

http://training.seer.cancer.gov/ss_module04_colon/unit02_sec01_anatomy

http://www.barcnetwork.org/i/biliarytract.png

http://scienceblogs.com

http://www.breastailments.com/structure.htm

http://www.hunterian.gla.ac.uk/collections/anatomy/students_projects/
spinalcord

http://www.montana.edu

http://www.yourdictionary.com

http://sickle.bwh.harvard.edu/fe-def.html

http://health.allrefer.com/pictures-images/throat-anatomy.html